Healing

Yourself:

A Nurse's

Guide to

Self-Care

and

Renewal

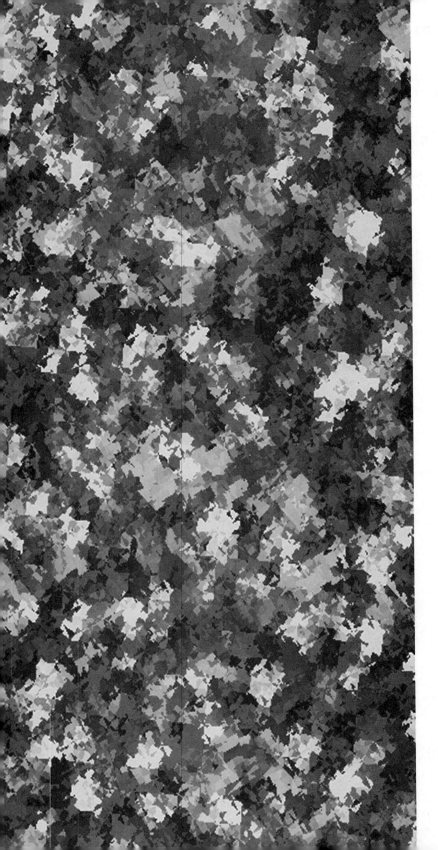

Healing Yourself:
A Nurse's Guide to Self-Care and Renewal

Sherry Kahn, MPH

Health Educator, Writer, Massage Therapist, and Director, *Self-Care for Caregivers*—in-house workshops and California mountain retreats. Ms. Kahn is also an experienced healthcare management consultant and trainer.

Mileva Saulo, EdD, RN

Assistant Professor, University of Southern California School of Nursing, and President, *Saulo and Associates*, a consulting practice specializing in organizational transformation. Dr. Saulo has an extensive background in undergraduate and graduate nursing education, nursing service administration, and professional nursing associations.

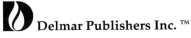

Delmar Publishers Inc. ™

I T P™

NOTICE TO THE READER

Publisher does not warrant or guarantee any of the products described herein or perform any independent analysis in connection with any of the product information contained herein. Publisher does not assume, and expressly disclaims, any obligation to obtain and include information other than that provided to it by the manufacturer.

The reader is expressly warned to consider and adopt all safety precautions that might be indicated by the activities described herein and to avoid all potential hazards. By following the instructions contained herein, the reader willingly assumes all risks in connection with such instructions.

The publisher makes no representations or warranties of any kind, including but not limited to, the warranties of fitness for particular purpose or merchantability, nor are any such representations implied with respect to the material set forth herein, and the publisher takes no responsibility with respect to such material. The publisher shall not be liable for any special, consequential or exemplary damages resulting, in whole or in part, from the readers' use of, or reliance upon, this material.

Cover Design: J^2 Designs

Delmar staff:
Publisher: David C. Gordon
Senior Acquisitions Editor: Bill Burgower
Assistant Editor: Debra M. Flis
Project Editor: Danya M. Plotsky
Production Coordinator: Barbara A. Bullock
Art and Design Coordinators: Megan K. Desantis
                                         Timothy J. Conners

For information, address

Delmar Publishers Inc.
3 Columbia Circle, Box 15015,
Albany, NY 12212-5015

Copyright © 1994 by Delmar Publishers Inc.

The trademark ITP is used under license.

Printed in the United States of America
Published simultaneously in Canada
by Nelson Canada,
a division of The Thomson Corporation

1 2 3 4 5 6 7 8 9 10 XXX 00 99 98 97 96 95 94

Library of Congress Cataloging-in-Publication Data

Kahn, Sherry.
    Healing yourself: a nurse's guide to self-care and renewal / Sherry Kahn, Mileva Saulo
        p. cm. — (RealNursing series)
    Includes index.
    ISBN 0-8273-6150-5
    1. Nursing—Psychological aspects. 2. Nurses—Job stress. 3. Burn out (Psychology)—Prevention.
    4. Stress Management.
    I. Saulo, Mileva. II. Title. III. Series.
    [DNLM: 1. Nursing. 2. Nurses—psychology. 3. Stress, Psychological—prevention & control—nurses'
    instruction. 4. Adaptation, Psychological—nurses' instruction. WY 87 K12h 1993]
RT86.K34 1993
610.73'01'9—dc20   93-26360
DNLM/DLC   CIP

RealNursing Series
Alice M. Stein, MA, RN, Series Editor
Medical College of Pennsylvania

Table of Contents

CHAPTER 8
BREATHING: THE ESSENCE OF LIFE ■ 87

CHAPTER 9
AEROBIC EXERCISE: THE ACTIVE FORM ■ 95

CHAPTER 10
YOGA ASANAS: THE RECEPTIVE FORM ■ 109

CHAPTER 11
MASSAGE: FOR HEALING AND RELAXATION ∎127

CHAPTER 12
SELF-MASSAGE: ACUPRESSURE ∎135

CHAPTER 13
SELF-MASSAGE: FOOT REFLEXOLOGY ∎151

CHAPTER 14
NUTRITION: THE BASICS ∎159

Preface

We live in a high-tech, low-touch era. This operational mode may have made us efficient, but it certainly has not made us healthy. As a nurse, your daily environment is a technological wonderland in which you are often caring for people who have succumbed to the stress diseases inherent in living in such a world. It is time for a paradigm shift from high-tech, low-touch to high-tech, high-touch. The first step in making that shift is to take care of yourself—to access the wonderful tools that have emerged from the wisdom of the east and the scientific acuity of the west.

Today, an evolution, rather than a revolution, is occurring in health-care in the United States. That evolution is toward wellness and self-responsibility. People are taking charge of their lives and their health at a time when so many factors in our external environment appear to be out of control.

In a landmark study recently published in *The New England Journal of Medicine*, it was reported that one in three individuals used some form of alternative medicine during the course of the preceding year. Most of this care was directed toward health promotion, disease prevention, or alleviation of uncomplicated conditions. When PBS aired its "Healing and the Mind" series, its audience was twice the number of the network's regular viewers, and the book of the same name is a bestseller. Even the federal government has taken notice of this trend toward alternative medicine and illness prevention, responding with the establishment of the Office for the Study of Unconventional Medical Practices at the National Institutes of Health.

Healing Yourself: A Nurse's Guide to Self-Care and Renewal is a compendium of some of the best information, exercises, and self-instructional techniques available for achieving and maintaining harmony of body, mind, and spirit. It is a convenient way for you to start developing a healthier, fuller you at your own pace and in your own space. As you learn new ways to manage your fast-moving world and renew yourself, you will be more capable of providing the high-touch caring that you and your patients, colleagues, family, and friends are so ready to receive.

The idea for this book came to co-author Sherry Kahn during a meditation. She expresses her gratitude to Spirit and to the Agape International Center of Truth for creating an appropriate atmosphere in which to receive and nurture the notion. The next layer of thanks goes to William Burgower, Senior Administrative Editor at Delmar and a holistic life-styler, for his openness and responsiveness to the idea and his continuing support during the writing of the book.

More thanks are in order from Sherry Kahn to Marguerite Baca, Jan Boller, Joyce Johnson, Katryne Koller, Haizen Paige, and Brenda Woods for providing information and support, and to all the people who and all the experiences which were her teachers.

Mileva Saulo expresses her gratitude to Dr. William Van Burgess, chair of her dissertation committee, who in the midst of chaos taught her to focus, to acknowledge the limits of her humanness, and to value success in small, measured steps; to Rev. Robert W. Howell, who helps her to see the miracles in life's stresses and transitions as opportunities for Spirit to come forward for new birth, again and again; to Geri Snider, who introduced her to transpersonal psychology, eastern thought, and nontraditional healing; to Irene Herrold, an octogenarian who teaches her that life is a continuous journey of growth and renewal; and to her mother, Catherine, and her late father, Michael, for supporting and nurturing her inclination to march to the tune of a different drummer and choose the road not taken.

And, finally, a word must be spoken for Yogi, the high-tech computer that made the efficient creation of this high-touch book possible.

Foreword

One advantage of getting older is to see certain ideas, ways of thinking, and trends come of age and other, older ideas resurface. In our time, both these phenomena have occurred, with the blending of Western and Eastern ways of thinking and the return of our own traditional values of caring. It is now widely accepted that the human aspects of care are as essential as the technological ones. More and more attention is devoted to humanizing the healthcare environment. An important part of this way of thinking is the recognition that the well-being and health of caregivers is critical to enhancing the care that they provide to their patients. The vision of the American Association of Critical-Care Nurses is that of *a healthcare system driven by the needs of patients in which healthcare providers make their optimal contribution*. We must do everything in our power to create systems that are centered on the needs of patients and support the caregivers in their efforts to provide optimal care. Part of that support is to promote the personal health and well-being of the care provider.

In his book *The 7 Habits of Highly Effective People*, Steven Covey talks about the importance of "sharpening the saw," that is, preserving and enhancing your greatest asset—you. He talks about the four dimensions of personal renewal: physical, mental, social/emotional, and spiritual. *Healing Yourself: A Nurse's Guide to Self-Care and Renewal* is a "how-to" approach for attending to yourself as a person so that you can make an optimal contribution in caring for your patients.

Years ago, when I was a critical-care clinical nurse educator, a colleague and I introduced weekly self-care sessions into our critical-care orientation program. The sessions were called "Pressure Adaptation" to make them sound as technical and as much like hemodynamic pressure monitoring as possible. We wondered if we could afford to take time out of the highly technical orientation to provide an hour a week for soft content focusing on stress reduction. To our pleasant surprise, that class became one of the highest rated sessions in the orientation program. We learned that it was well worth the investment in time to devote a portion of the curriculum to personal renewal and balance. The sessions were held each Friday, and the new employees left for the weekend refreshed, energized, and uplifted. You could feel the tensions disappear and the moods elevate. Several of the topics we covered in that class are presented in this book.

In reviewing *Healing Yourself: A Nurse's Guide to Self-Care and Renewal,* I experienced many of the same feelings of renewal and relaxation that I had in my classes. My mood turned from overburdened to positive. I exercised more and ate better. I had more energy. I believe that every caregiver should have access to a book like this both at home and at work. Each chapter is brief and provides a good overview of different aspects of attending to the self. The content is relevant for curricula in academic, staff development, and continuing education settings, and useful for experts as well as novices.

I know that the authors "walk the talk" of this guide. And I look forward to the outcomes of their intent in writing this book—to highly dedicated health professionals who care for themselves as well as they care for their patients.

Jan Boller, RN, MSN
Program Development Director
American Association of Critical-Care Nurses

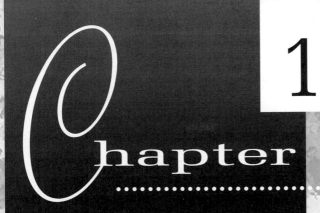

Chapter 1

The Nurse as Caregiver

PROFESSIONAL CAREGIVER

As a nurse, you have chosen a career as a professional caregiver. Your lifework is a noble one, that of nurturing, nourishing, and caring for those in need. Your responsibilities may vary from routine care to tending to the acutely or critically ill, but typically you are on the front lines every day.

You are in intimate contact with your patients, providing not only physical support but emotional nurturance as well. During the course of a year you may be involved with hundreds, even thousands, of sick and needy individuals, each requiring specialized treatment. For those without or alienated from relatives and friends, you may be their only personal contact.

Not only are you essential to your patients' well-being, you are an important member of a larger group of caregivers. That multidisciplinary team includes physicians, physical therapists, social workers, dieticians, laboratory technicians, respiratory therapists, orderlies, receptionists, and many other skilled workers needed to deliver the high quality, high-tech healthcare we all rely upon.

THE DEMANDS OF NURSING

Nursing is a very worthy but demanding profession that calls upon its members for the ultimate form of giving—altruism, the unselfish caring for others. Most individuals who select nursing as a career have a desire to give to others, to provide care and comfort, to relieve pain and suffering, and ultimately, to make a difference in the lives of people in need. And nurses do all these things daily.

Ongoing demands of patients, superiors, and coworkers can, however, create stress even for the hardiest of nurses. This stress can come from many sources—long shifts, large patient loads, needy patients, ethical dilemmas, unpleasant coworkers, controlling superiors, cumbersome bureaucracy, inadequate facilities and supplies, and so on. Your personal life may also, either intermittently or consistently, be another source of stress.

THE NURSE AS SELF-NURTURER

Those who choose the helping professions often have an easier time giving to others than giving to themselves. In fact, many professional helpers do not know how to care for themselves. The reasons for this are myriad, ranging from religious beliefs to a dysfunctional family background to the ways in which women are socialized. Regardless of the reasons, the results are the same. Caregivers who do not nurture themselves sooner or later manifest stress symptoms and diseases. Some are mild, such as headaches or backaches; others, such as heart disease and cancer, are life-threatening.

TOOLS FOR THE CAREGIVER

Tools for Managing Stress

Since stress is and will continue to be a part of your nursing life, the key to your survival and to enjoying your career is learning how to manage stress.

In the last forty years extensive research has been conducted on the causes of stress and the development of tools for managing it. The last few decades have seen scientific documentation in the West of many valuable stress management techniques that have been practiced in the East for millenniums. Large strides have been made as well in understanding child and adult psychology and the psychology of addictions. Today we are truly fortunate to have not only this knowledge of mind, body, and spirit but also practical ways to apply it in our everyday lives.

Tools for Personal Renewal

Humans have an innate need for positive change and growth. The same knowledge that can be used for stress management may also be used for personal renewal. Once you have learned how to manage stress in your life, you can use the resulting freed energy to realize the fullness of your creativity and joyfulness.

USING YOUR TOOLCHEST

This book is your personal toolchest for managing stress and enjoying personal renewal. In it you will find ways to bring yourself into and maintain balance in mind, body, and spirit. Giving from this holistic state of harmony is a different experience—a fulfilling one rather than a depleting one.

We begin with a look at stress—its physiology, causes, and effects. Next we look at the mind: first, the emotions that can create stress or be a reaction to stress and then the thought process and how to use thoughts to modify your experience. Then we move to connection with the spirit and the disciplines of meditation and breathing. From there, we proceed to focus on the body and on how the proper use of exercise (aerobics and yoga), nutrition, and self-massage can reduce stress and enhance growth. We conclude with a look at some additional tools for positive transformation and the process of change.

Self-evaluation forms are included in key chapters to help you identify aspects of your attitudes, beliefs, and behaviors of which you may be unaware. Diagrams are provided to assist you with yoga postures and self-massage, and clear and simple directions are provided for a variety of self-help activities.

Since this book is designed as a self-care resource, each section is independent of the others. For example, you may use the section on emotions or nutrition without reading the surrounding material.

ONE STEP AT A TIME

Our purpose here is to offer a variety of techniques for stress reduction, health maintenance, and personal renewal. We suggest that you not try to do everything at once. That in itself can be very stressful! Instead, select one area that you feel would be most beneficial to you, is fairly easy for you to incorporate into your life-style, and is something you would enjoy doing. As you master one area, move on to another. Remember, this book is your personal toolchest. Use and enjoy it.

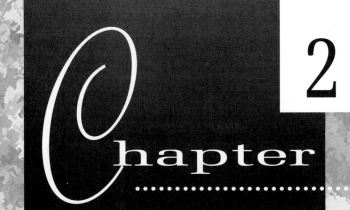

Chapter 2

Stress

WHAT IS STRESS?

Stress is strain or pressure from an external trigger that can produce physiological and emotional responses. The majority of visits to physicians are for stress-related problems, which may express themselves in a variety of symptoms as shown in Figure 2-1.

FIGURE 2-1
COMMON SYMPTOMS OF STRESS

Headache	Insomnia
Backache	Dizziness/faintness
Fatigue	Increased blood pressure
Constipation	Jaw clenching
Diarrhea	Heart palpitations
Nausea/vomiting	Agitation
Intestinal distress	Shakiness
Loss of appetite	Irritability
Compulsive eating	Worry
Breathlessness	Inability to concentrate
Cold hands or feet	Forgetfulness
Oversleeping	Panic

PHYSIOLOGY OF STRESS

Since the brain and the nervous system are so intimately involved in stress reactions, a quick review of these systems is useful for understanding the research in this area.

The brain controls two nervous systems in the body: the central nervous system (CNS) and the autonomic nervous system (ANS). The CNS is responsible for the capacity to walk, talk, and perform gross and fine muscle movements. The ANS is responsible for control of bodily functions that are not consciously directed, including regular beating of the heart, breathing, intestinal movements, perspiration, salivation, and so on.

The ANS is subdivided into the sympathetic and the parasympathetic nervous systems. The interplay of sympathetic and parasympathetic reflexes governs their activities. The sympathetic system increases blood pressure and the pace of breathing, causes sweating, cools the skin, and activates the production of sugar. The parasympathetic reaction is opposite to that of the sympathetic system. Thus the parasympathetic system decreases the heart rate, slows breathing, retards perspiration, and accelerates stomach and gastrointestinal activity. It is the sympathetic nervous system that is activated in response to stress.

The Fight or Flight Response

The discovery of stress as a physiological state is a result of the pioneering work of the Hungarian physician Dr. Hans Selye (Selye, Note 1). Selye divided stress into two categories, *eustress* and *distress*. He defined eustress as good stress, such as that involved in falling in love or buying a new house. Distress was defined as bad stress, of the sort experienced when facing the threat of physical injury. Both types of stress produce similar physiological responses brought about by the stimulation of the sympathetic nervous system. Selye called these responses the *General Adaptation Syndrome.*

The body becomes charged with energy either to stay and fight or to take off in flight. As Selye noted, this response was an essential instinctive survival mechanism for our primitive ancestors, who were often faced with real physical danger.

As the body responds to stress, the adrenal glands pump adrenaline, comprised of the two hormones, norepinephrine and epinephrine, into the bloodstream for added strength. Norepinephrine has its greatest effect in increasing the heart rate and blood pressure. Epinephrine has its greatest effect in releasing stored sugar for use as energy. Additional hormones, corticosteroids, also secreted in reaction to a stressor, trigger the release of fatty acids into the blood.

During a prolonged state of arousal, as happens with distress, the body moves from a state of combat readiness into a state of diminishing return. The corticosteroids, designed to reduce inflammation and tissue injury during the fight stage, will over a prolonged period of activation suppress the functioning of the immune system. High corticosteroid levels can also contribute to stomach ulcerations caused by increased acid formation and to a decrease in lean muscle due to its consumption as an energy source.

The increased amounts of fatty acids circulating in the blood are converted to cholesterol by the liver and can thus potentially lead to arteriosclerosis. The accelerated heart rate needed to circulate oxygen and body chemicals rapidly during situations calling for a quick response increases the risks of hypertension, stroke, and heart disease. The combined action of adrenaline and corticosteroids blocks the action of insulin, thereby increasing the availability of blood sugar for immediate needs—so continually high levels of these hormones may also aggravate diabetes.

Daily Stress Reactions

Just about everyone has experienced, at one time or another, the extreme fight or flight response just described. However, each of us may in the routine of our daily lives experience as many as 20 to 50 small emotional arousals that trigger a stress reaction, reports Dr. Keith Sedlacek, medical director of the Stress Regulation Institute in New York (Sedlacek, Note 2). The daily worries of modern life can keep the mind in a state of fear and anxiety and the body in a state of activation and physiological stress.

These reactions, which may even occur during sleep, produce slight increases in heart rate and blood pressure, and also muscle tightening. These continued arousals can have a cumulative effect, leading to such stress symptoms as headaches, backaches, digestive disturbances, eating disorders, and sleep disturbance.

One way to become aware of your daily stresses and your reactions to them is to keep a log. Figure 2-2 is a useful self-monitoring tool for this purpose. If copied and used every day for one week, both at work and at home, it will provide you with a pattern of your stress symptoms, the types of activities or interactions that stress you, what emotions and thoughts these stress responses generate, and how you react to each stressful situation.

For example, you may find that you get a headache every time you interact with a particular type of patient, that this creates a feeling of anger and impatience in you, and that your response is to take an aspirin and ignore your feelings. Or you may experience stomach agitation and nervousness when your least favorite relative calls, and your response may be to play a calming piece of music after you hang up.

According to Selye, continual reactions to stress over a long time period deplete the body of available energy and accelerate natural aging and deterioration. Selye labeled this third and final phase of the General Adaptation Syndrome the *stage of exhaustion*. Traditional Chinese medicine holds a similar view. The Chinese call the body's inborn vital energy supply *jing*. Jing is stored in the kidney area—the

FIGURE 2-2
Daily Stress Log

Date:_____ Day of Week:_____

TIME OF DAY	WHERE	PHYSICAL SYMPTOM(S)	EVENT/ACTIVITY

PERSON(S) INVOLVED	THOUGHTS/FEELINGS	RESPONSE TO STRESS

site of the adrenals—and becomes depleted with unhealthy living. East Indians call this vital force *prana* and prescribe ways to prevent its depletion.

New research confirms these views, relating persistent unrelenting stress reactions to significant distortions in the body's natural balance. These chronic physiological disturbances, in turn, lead to characteristic diseases of premature aging and deterioration such as cancer, heart disease, and musculoskeletal degeneration.

Psychoneuroimmunology

The new and exciting area of research called *psychoneuroimmunology* (PNI) looks at the interrelationships among the mind (psychology), the brain (neurology), and the body's natural healing system (immunology).

Three communication systems link the mind and the body: the CNS, the ANS, and the neuropeptide chemical messenger system. The operation of the CNS and ANS was summarized earlier in this chapter. The neuropeptide chemical messenger system is the most recently discovered link between the mind and the body.

Research at Johns Hopkins University led to the discovery that brain cells have receptors for specific chemicals and that the body naturally produces chemicals to fit these receptors (Pert, Note 3). These chemicals are *neuropeptides*, basic amino acid peptide chains produced in the brain. The first neuropeptide discovered was beta-endorphin, an internal morphine. Since then an additional 50 to 60 neuropeptides have been identified.

It is now known that neuropeptides are produced not only in the brain but by cells throughout the body, including the hormonal and immune cells. The brain communicates to the body chemically, and the body is able to communicate back to the brain in the same manner.

Hormonal cells release hormones, activate physiological functions, and maintain a steady-state environment in the body. Immune cells identify and destroy viruses, bacteria, and abnormal cells, heal wounds, and are also responsible for maintaining homeostasis. The health and well-being of the body are dependent upon the optimal functioning of both the hormonal and immune systems.

These systems are directly influenced by mental states. It has now been shown that neuropeptide synthesis is activated by positive feelings and thoughts and by the attitudes of joy, peace, confidence, and love. Negative states such as stress, helplessness, depression, hostility, and anger suppress neuropeptide production.

RELATIONSHIP OF STRESS TO HEALTH

Negative reactions to stress have a direct impact on our physiology, our risk of developing life-threatening diseases related to compromised immune and hormonal systems, and ultimately our longevity. Recent research clearly demonstrates the causal relationship between stress and ill health.

Stress Research

It has been observed that when one spouse in a long-term marriage dies it is not uncommon for the remaining spouse to die shortly thereafter. Researchers at Mount Sinai School of Medicine were able to document an actual, detectable suppression of the immune system during the bereavement period in men whose wives had recently died (Schleiffer & Keller, Note 4).

A series of experiments performed on medical students demonstrated that the stressful event of taking examinations resulted in measurable suppression of immune system-related values in their blood samples (Kiecolt-Glaser et al, Note 5). Other studies in the workplace found that individuals with highly demanding jobs who perceived that they had little control over their work had three times the average probability of developing high blood pressure and a substantially increased incidence of structural damage to the heart (Schnall, Note 6).

The nature of the herpes virus provides another source of evidence of the relationship between stress and poor health. The herpes virus remains in the body for the lifetime of the individual infected, and whether it is active or dormant depends on the competence of the individual's immune system. Active eruptions have been shown to be related to stress, unhappiness, marital disruption, and student test taking (Kiecolt-Glaser & Glaser, Note 7).

The Power of Perceptions

Some of the most interesting PNI findings concern the relationship among conditioning, perceptions, and physiological reactions. One of the breakthrough studies in this field was a negative conditioning experiment conducted on rats. In an effort to cause the rats to develop an aversion to saccharine, they were injected with a nausea producing drug before they drank sweetened water. Usually, after just one injection of the drug the rats conditioned themselves to feel nauseous on tasting the sweetened water. However, the most surprising result of this study was that the rats died shortly afterward. It turned out that the nausea producing drug was also a strong immunosuppressant and that the rats had, in effect, conditioned themselves to suppress their immune systems (Barber, Note 8).

A dramatic illustration of the power of perception on health outcome was reported by Dr. Deepak Chopra, a practicing endocrinologist, former chief of staff of New England Memorial Hospital, and one of the foremost leaders in PNI. A patient dying of cancer was given one dose of an experimental drug at a time when it was believed he only had a few days to live. His tumors rapidly decreased in size beyond all expectations, and his vitality returned. The patient then read a news report claiming the ineffectiveness of the drug and quickly relapsed. His physician gave him a double dose of the drug and the patient rebounded dramatically. Shortly thereafter another news account reported that the drug the patient had been given had been found to be totally worthless. Within days the patient grew despondent, the tumors enlarged, and he died several days later.

Norman Cousins, another PNI pioneer who demonstrated the connection between the mind and the body by healing his own "incurable" disease, observed many patient perception reactions. He noted numerous instances of sudden decreases in immune function when patients were told by their physicians that their condition was terminal or hopeless.

Chopra and Cousins also describe many cases of apparently "miraculous" recoveries of terminal patients that seemed to have been linked to their beliefs. The immune system appears to "know" how we think and feel, is affected by our general mental state, and in turn, communicates back to our mind, resulting in subsequent health or disease. This relationship has led to the coining of the term *bodymind* by those who, in essence, view the body and mind as a unified entity and not as two separate, unrelated objects.

YOUR PERSONAL STRESSORS

Everyone has stressors in their lives. Some people have more than others, and some people adapt to stress better than do others. Being aware of the stressors in your life and of the amount of stress you are experiencing can be a powerful motivator for taking positive action.

Developed by Dr. Thomas Holmes and Dr. Richard Rahe at the University of Washington School of Medicine, the Social Readjustment Rating Scale is still employed as an objective way of measuring stress exposure over a period of one year. The scale includes both eustress items such as vacation, outstanding personal achievement, and Christmas, and distress items such as problems with work, marriage, and so forth.

The Social Readjustment Rating Scale, shown in Figure 2-3, is included here for your use. Take a few minutes to answer each item and total your score.

FIGURE 2-3
The Social Readjustment Rating Scale
••

Directions: Read each Life Event and indicate in the space provided the number of times you have experienced the event in the last year. Multiply the number of times you experienced the event by the points next to it and total up the products.

Life Event	Stress Value	Number of times you experienced the event last year	Your total life changes scores
1. Death of spouse	100 x	_____ =	_____
2. Divorce	73 x	_____ =	_____
3. Marital separation from mate	65 x	_____ =	_____
4. Detention in jail or other institution	63 x	_____ =	_____
5. Death of a close family member	63 x	_____ =	_____
6. Major personal injury or illness	53 x	_____ =	_____
7. Marriage	50 x	_____ =	_____
8. Being fired from work	47 x	_____ =	_____
9. Marital reconciliation with mate	45 x	_____ =	_____
10. Retirement from work	45 x	_____ =	_____
11. Major change in the health or behavior of a family member	44 x	_____ =	_____
12. Pregnancy	40 x	_____ =	_____
13. Sexual difficulties	39 x	_____ =	_____

14. Gaining a new family member (e.g through birth, adoption, oldster moving in, etc.) ....39 x _____ = _____

15. Major business readjustment (e.g. merger, reorganization, bankruptcy, etc.)...............................39 x _____ = _____

16. Major change in financial state (e.g. a lot worse off or a lot better off than usual)..............................38 x _____ = _____

17. Death of a close friend ....37 x _____ = _____

18. Changing to a different line of work.........................36 x _____ = _____

19. Major change in the number of arguments with spouse (e.g. either a lot more or a lot less than usual regarding childbearing, personal habits, etc.)...............35 x _____ = _____

20. Purchasing a home, business, etc. ....31 x _____ = _____

21. Foreclosure on a mortgage or loan ....30 x _____ = _____

22. Major change in responsibilities at work (e.g. promotion, demotion, lateral transfer) ....29 x _____ = _____

23. Son or daughter leaving home (e.g. marriage, attending college, etc.) ....29 x _____ = _____

24. Inlaw troubles...29 x _____ = _____

25. Outstanding personal achievement............................28 x _____ = _____

26. Wife beginning or ceasing working outside the home ....26 x _____ = _____

27. Beginning or ceasing formal schooling ....26 x _____ = _____

28. Major change in living conditions (e.g. building a new home, remodeling, deterioration of home or neighborhood)..25 x _____ = _____

29. Revision of personal habits (e.g. dress, manners, associations, etc.) ....24 x _____ = _____

30. Troubles with the boss...23 x _____ = _____

31. Major change in working hours or conditions......................20 x _____ = _____

32. Change in residence...20 x _____ = _____

33. Changing to a new school...20 x _____ = _____

34. Major change in usual type and/or amount of recreation ......19 x _____ = _____

35. Major change in church activities (e.g. a lot more or a lot less than usual)..19 x _____ = _____

36. Major change in social activities (e.g. clubs, dancing, movies, visiting, etc.) ....19 x _____ = _____

37. Taking on a loan less than $10,000 ....17 x _____ = _____

38. Major change in sleeping habits (e.g. a lot more or a
    lot less sleep, or change in part of day when asleep) ....16 x _____ = _____

39. Major change in number of family get-togethers
    (e.g. a lot more or a lot less than usual)....................................15 x _____ = _____

40. Major change in eating habits (e.g. a lot more or a lot less
    food intake, or very different meal hours, or surroundings)..15 x _____ = _____

41. Vacation...13 x _____ = _____

42. Christmas...12 x _____ = _____

43. Minor violations of the law (e.g. traffic tickets,
    jaywalking, disturbing the peace, etc.)....................................11 x _____ = _____

    GRAND TOTAL ...._____

Adapted and reprinted with permission from the *Journal of Psychosomatic Research*, *2*, Holmes, T.H. and Rahe. "The Social Readjustment Rating Scale"© 1967, Pergamon Press, Ltd.

A score of 150 to 300 is considered moderate, while a score of 300 or more is considered high. The higher the score, the greater is the susceptibility to illnesses or accidents. If you scored high, it does not necessarily mean that you are heading for a disaster. What it does mean is that you have experienced considerable stress in the past year.

Now that you have this awareness, you can choose to respond in one of two ways. You can decide to ignore it and hope that your strong genetic constitution will carry you through, or you can choose to start practicing some stress reduction techniques to reduce your risk.

PERSONALTITY TYPES AND STRESS

Another way to assess your personal relationship with stress is to examine your personality type. Dr. Meyer Friedman and Dr. Ray Rosenman conducted a 12-year study of 3,500 men that resulted in the publication of *Type A Behavior and Your Health* (Friedman & Rosenman, Note 9). Each man was classified as either Type A or Type B based on a number of personality characteristics. This and other personality paradigms are useful in assessing your probable reaction to stress.

Type A

The Type A personality is aggressive and involved in an incessant struggle to achieve more in less time. Type A people are also typically hostile to others. They always walk, move, talk, and eat quickly. Finishing others' sentences and interrupting are other commonly observed Type A behaviors.

Type A individuals are extremely competitive. Their goals are to have more of everything—possessions, activities, and friends. They are achievement oriented, judging themselves by the number rather than the quality of their successes.

Physically, Type As often exhibit "struggle" gestures such as grinding their teeth or clenching their fists, and their bodies are in a chronic state of stress. Because of their constantly high levels of adrenalin and corticosteroids, Type A individuals show increased cholesterol and fat levels in their bloodstream as well as increased clotting in the arteries.

The study results showed, not surprisingly, that the Type A participants were two to three times more prone to heart attacks than their Type B conterparts who did not exhibit these behavior patterns.

Hostility, now recognized as one of the most powerful triggers of stress reactions, plays a potent role in increasing the risk of heart disease. A study of 118 lawyers over a 25-year period showed that those Type As who tested high in hostility as law students had a mortality rate due to heart disease over four times greater than their more relaxed peers (Williams, Note 10).

Type As are typically self-involved, using "I" and "me" much more frequently than Type Bs. Individuals with this pattern of excessive self-involvement were also found to have increased blood pressure levels and anger intensity (Scherwitz et al, Note 11).

Type B

Type B individuals are much more relaxed than Type As. They tend to be patient and lack a driving sense of urgency. They usually do one thing at a time rather than several. They enjoy the process of what they are doing for its own sake rather than solely for the end result of accomplishment.

Type Bs are easygoing, good listeners, and enjoy their recreation time.

Typing Yourself

Some people can easily identify with either the Type A or Type B personality. Many people, however, exhibit some characteristics of both. Figure 2-4 provides you with an opportunity to see where you fall on the A–B Scale.

FIGURE 2-4
THE A/B LIFE-STYLE QUESTIONNAIRE

Directions: As you can see, each scale below is composed of a pair of adjectives or phrases. Each pair represents two kinds of contrasting behavior. Choose the number that most closely represents the type of person you are and put it under the column labeled YOUR SCORE. Add your scores to get your total score.

RATING SCALE

YOUR SCORE

1.	Work regular hours	0 1 2 3 4 5 6 7 8 9 10	Bring work home or work late	_____
2.	Wait calmly	0 1 2 3 4 5 6 7 8 9 10	Wait impatiently	_____
3.	Seldom judge in terms of numbers (how many, how much)	0 1 2 3 4 5 6 7 8 9 10	Place value in terms of numbers	_____
4.	Not competitive	0 1 2 3 4 5 6 7 8 9 10	Very competitive	_____
5.	Feel limited responsibility	0 1 2 3 4 5 6 7 8 9 10	Always feel responsible	_____
6.	Unhurried about appointments	0 1 2 3 4 5 6 7 8 9 10	Frequently hurried for appointments	_____
7.	Never in a hurry	0 1 2 3 4 5 6 7 8 9 10	Always in a hurry	_____
8.	Many interests	0 1 2 3 4 5 6 7 8 9 10	Work is main interest	_____
9.	Try to satisfy self	0 1 2 3 4 5 6 7 8 9 10	Want to be recognized by others	_____
10.	Not very precise	0 1 2 3 4 5 6 7 8 9 10	Careful about detail	_____
11.	Can leave things temporarily unfinished	0 1 2 3 4 5 6 7 8 9 10	Must get things finished	_____
12.	Satisfied with job	0 1 2 3 4 5 6 7 8 9 10	Striving on the job	_____
13.	Listen well	0 1 2 3 4 5 6 7 8 9 10	Finish sentences for others	_____
14.	Easygoing	0 1 2 3 4 5 6 7 8 9 10	Hard driving	_____
15.	Do things slowly	0 1 2 3 4 5 6 7 8 9 10	Do things quickly	_____
16.	Do one thing at a time	0 1 2 3 4 5 6 7 8 9 10	Think about what to do next	_____
17.	Rarely angry	0 1 2 3 4 5 6 7 8 9 10	Easily angered	_____
18.	Slow speech	0 1 2 3 4 5 6 7 8 9 10	Forceful speech	_____
19.	Express feelings easily	0 1 2 3 4 5 6 7 8 9 10	Bottle up feelings	_____
20.	Rarely set deadlines	0 1 2 3 4 5 6 7 8 9 10	Often set deadlines	_____

YOUR TOTAL A/B SCORE   _____

A total score of less than 100 reflects a relaxed behavior that exhibits few of the reactions associated with heart disease. A total score of 100–134 shows a mixture of A and B behaviors. A total score in the 135–159 range puts you in the position of being prone to cardiac problems. If your total is 160–200 you have a very high heart disease risk, particularly if you are over 40 years of age and smoke.

Type C

Looking at the extremes of the aggressive, competitive Type A and the relaxed, low-key Type B, two psychologists, Dr. Robert Kriegel and Dr. Marilyn Harris Kriegel, felt that there was something less than optimal in both types. Type A performs well under the pressures of modern life but pays the price for it. Type B, although easygoing and healthier than Type A, lacks the spark, the enthusiasm, the excitement of life.

Observing peak performers in the arenas of sports and business, the Kriegels defined a new behavior type, which they called Type C. Type C behavior is peak performance under pressure without the debilitating effects of stress. In the Type C behavior mode, performance is effortless, and the individual is more effective and productive than usual, focused and spontaneous, and filled with vitality.

Behavioral characteristics most frequently mentioned by people who function regularly in this mode are confidence, commitment, and control. Practicing some of the techniques in this book—mindcise, meditation, and yoga (Chapters 6, 7, and 10)—will assist you in achieving these optimal performance characteristics.

INTERRUPTING THE CYCLE

Unlike our primitive ancestors who were unable to differentiate between perceived and real threats to their survival, you have the ability to discern what is really happening when your body has a stress reaction or manifests a stress symptom.

As soon as you become aware that you are having a stress reaction, stop, evaluate your situation, and interrupt the stress cycle. For example, if you find yourself with your muscles tensing as you react to a physician's unreasonable demands, stop and analyze the situation. Responding with a workable compromise, rather than reacting as if you had no choice, is a healthy way to interrupt your stress reaction.

Taking a proactive approach—choosing a health-promoting response—rather than simply reacting to a situation is a valuable stress survival tool. The breathing, meditation, and mindcise techniques described in Chapter 6, 7, and 8 can facilitate your ability to move quickly from a reactive to a proactive position.

NOTES

1. Selye, H. *The Stress of Life*, rev. ed., New York: McGraw-Hill Book Co., 1976.

2. Sedlacek, K. *The Sedlacek Technique: Finding the Calm Within You*, New York: McGraw-Hill Book Co., 1989.

3. Pert, C. The wisdom of the receptors: neuropeptides, the emotions and bodymind. *Advances, Institute for the Advancement of Health, 3*, 1986, 3.

4. Schleiffer, S.J. and Keller, S.E., et al. Suppression of lymphocyte stimulation during bereavement. *JAMA*, 1983, *250*, 374.

5. Kiecolt-Glaser, J. et al. Psychological modifiers of immunocompetence in medical students. *Psychosomatic Medicine*, 1984, *46*, 1.

6. Schnall, P.L. The relationship between "job strain" in workplace diastolic blood pressure and left ventricular mass index. *JAMA*, 1990, *263*, 1929.

7. Kiecolt-Glaser, J. and Glaser, R. Psychological influences on immunity. *American Psychologist*, Nov. 1988.

8. Barber, J. Worried sick. *Equinox*, 1988, *108*, 91–93.

9. Friedman, M. and Rosenman, R. *Type A Behavior and Your Health*, New York: Alfred A. Knopf, 1974.

10. Williams, R. *The Trusting Heart*, New York: Springer Publishing Company, 1988.

11. Scherwitz, L., Graham, L. E. II and Ornish, D. Self-involvement and the risk factors for coronary heart disease, *Advances*, 1985, *2*, 6-18.

SELECTED BIBLIOGRAPHY

Borysenko, J. *Minding the Body, Mending the Mind*. New York: Bantam Books, 1987.

Charlesworth, E. A. and Nathan, R. G. *Stress Management: A Comprehensive Guide to Wellness*. New York: Atheneum, 1984.

Chopra, D. *Quantum Healing: Exploring the Frontiers of Mind/Body Medicine*. New York: Bantam Books, 1990.

Cousins, N. *Head First: The Biology of Hope and the Healing Power of the Human Spirit*. New York: Penguin, 1989.

Dacher, E. S. *PNI: Psychoneuroimmunology: The New Mind/Body Healing Program*. New York: Paragon House, 1990.

Kriegel, R. J. and Kriegel, M. H. *The C Zone: Peak Performance Under Pressure*. Garden City, N. J.: Anchor Press/Doubleday, 1984.

Pelliter, K. *Mind as Healer, Mind as Slayer*. New York: Dell Books, 1977.

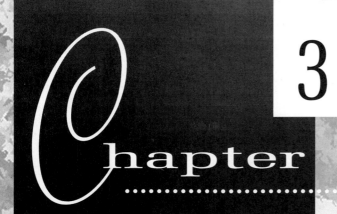

Chapter 3

Emotional Reactions in Nursing

THE EMOTIONAL DEMANDS OF NURSING

A certain set of characteristics typify the professional nursing role. As a nurse you are always expected to be kind, caring, patient, giving, calm, and respectful. At the same time you are supposed to be "professional"—responsible, intelligent, objective, and a rational decision-maker. Or, if you received your nursing training some years ago, you were taught that being professional meant being nonemotional and detached from your patients.

No matter how professional you act, nursing, by its very nature, is an emotionally demanding profession. As a nurse you provide not only physical but also emotional support for your patients. You are intimately involved with needy people all day long. Your days are often filled with patients suffering from painful, debilitating conditions; anxious, and sometimes hysterical, relatives and friends; and people who die no matter what you do.

As a nurse and a human you have feelings and experience emotional reactions to your environment. You may feel grief or depression when an infant dies, or guilt when your unit is understaffed and in your haste you make a medication error that creates difficulty for your patient. You may feel helpless or confused when a patient's family asks about the prognosis and you know that the physician has not been truthful with them. Feelings of anger or frustration may engulf you when your supervisor denies that a colleague who has shown up for work intoxicated is impaired in any way.

Guilt

Guilt is the feeling that springs from the conviction that "things would have been different if I had ..." or "I should have done...differently." For example, "If only I had gotten to Mr. Smeal's bed five minutes earlier, he would still be alive," or, "I know I should have changed the catheter on Mrs. Blevin, but I was busy with six other patients."

The reality is that you cannot change the past. What is past is past. But you can change the present and the future. The other reality is that we all make mistakes. You are human like everyone else, and to be human is to err from time to time.

You may have made a mistake, or you may simply have tried to be responsible for something that was not your responsibility. It really does not matter. The solution and the resolution are the same: you need to forgive yourself and release the emotion.

Depression

Depression can result from one particularly traumatic event or from a series of events that have a cumulative effect. If a patient you have been close to for months dies, your reaction to the event may be depression. Working on an AIDS unit, where the patients continuously die, can over a period of time lead you into a chronic state of despair.

The counteraction to feeling down or enervated is pleasurable activity. You cannot change what is happening to the patients for whom you are caring, but you can change what is happening to you. If you get depressed, either acutely or chronically, do something nice for yourself. Take a bubble bath, play a favorite piece of music, share time with joyous friends—do whatever makes you feel that there is good in the world and in your life. Depression is a state of stagnation. Create movement. Create change. Exercise is an effective antidote for depression. You cannot stay depressed while running.

Emotional Exhaustion

Emotional exhaustion is insidious. It creeps up on you gradually, bit by bit. Then, it seems that all of a sudden you have lost your sense of humor, you have become irritable, a small slight sends you into uncontrollable crying, and you begin to dislike your patients and your coworkers.

Emotional exhaustion is a state of imbalance. You are giving out more than you are taking in. In essence, your battery loses its charge. There is no circulation of current, and you become exhausted.

Nurturance is the remedy for emotional exhaustion. You need people to give to you and you need to give to yourself. If you do not have a support group for yourself, create one. It need not be an organized group. A few close friends who are really there for you and care about you unconditionally will serve you well. You also need to nurture yourself. Do your favorite things. Be kind and gentle with yourself. Explore some of the ways to provide care that are less taxing on you emotionally. The idea of "cognitive caring," discussed in detail in Chapter 5, and specific techniques for nurturing yourself presented in subsequent chapters are good starting points.

IMPORTANCE OF EMOTIONAL CLARITY

Because of the strongly interpersonal nature of your work, it is very important that you understand who you are emotionally. Each of us has emotional patterns that we carry with us from both childhood and adult experiences. Some of these are healthy and others are not so healthy. Some of the patterns that may have been useful for surviving a less than perfect childhood, for example, may be detrimental to you in your caregiving work. Identifying these patterns and releasing the negative ones are important steps in maintaining the healthy emotional balance you need to function well at work and to enjoy your life.

DYSFUNCTIONAL FAMILIES

What exactly is a dysfunctional family? A dysfunctional family is one in which the child's personal developmental needs are not met. As a result, the child does not develop a healthy inner life and grows into an adult who does not know his true self. It is estimated that the majority of today's adults—some experts say as many as 90%—grew up in dysfunctional families.

When natural child development stages are arrested or distorted, the child becomes an adult with an injured or incapacitated child inside. This inner child contaminates the adult, resulting in behaviors that are less than optimal, and sometimes extremely damaging, for a healthy adult life.

Dysfunctional families are the result of dysfunctional adults. If a mother and father are carrying inside themselves angry and hurt five-year-olds, they will have difficulty in providing the unconditional love, support, and nurturance that a child requires. The cycle continues from one generation to the next. Adults who were not properly nurtured as children fail to nurture their own children well, and these children grow up to become adults who in turn do not know how to provide for the healthy development of their children. Child abusers who themselves were abused children are an extreme manifestation of this pattern.

One classic example of a dysfunctional family is the alcoholic family in which one or both parents are chemically dependent on alcohol. In this type of family system, the members who do not drink become hypervigilant because the alcoholic's drinking is so threatening to the family's survival. When children are focused on survival and on being a parent to their parent, they often do not have the necessary time for their own inner development.

Another example of an unhealthy developmental environment is the situation where the child is made into a surrogate spouse. Instead of working on fixing or resolving their adult relationships, parents in bad marriages often look to their children to fulfill the emotional needs that are not being met by their spouses. The children caught in such situations grow up very confused about relationships with the opposite sex and about who they are as persons.

Figure 3-1 contains a series of questions that assess the extent to which your inner child may be injured. Taking a few minutes to answer these questions honestly will be very helpful in your understanding of your emotional patterning. Answer "yes" or "no" to each question.

FIGURE 3-1
Injured Child Questionnaire

	Yes	No	
1.	___	___	Do I feel like I have no identity of my own?
2.	___	___	Is pleasing others more important than pleasing myself?
3.	___	___	Do I feel that I am not really "all right"?
4.	___	___	Do I hold onto people, things, and feelings for a long time?
5.	___	___	Do I feel that I was never loved by one or both of my parents?
6.	___	___	Do I feel fearful or anxious whenever I think about doing something I have not done before?
7.	___	___	Do I tend to give in to others rather than standing firm in what I believe?
8.	___	___	Do I frequently criticize myself?
9.	___	___	Do I often feel depressed?
10.	___	___	Do I consider myself a perfectionist?
11.	___	___	Do I consider myself a superachiever or workaholic?
12.	___	___	Do I almost never express unpleasant emotions like fear, anger, shame, or guilt?
13.	___	___	Do I feel inadequate sexually?
14.	___	___	Do I experience addictive behavior with food, drugs, alcohol or sex, or I am married or emotionally involved with someone who expresses such addictive behaviors?
15.	___	___	Do I do anything to avoid being by myself?
16.	___	___	Even though I do not say "no" directly, do I avoid doing things I do not want to do by engaging in passive or manipulative behaviors?

       Yes No

17. ____ ____ Is my response to conflict to either withdraw or try to control the person with whom I am having difficulty?

18. ____ ____ Am I terrified of being abandoned in an intimate relationship and tend to hold on even when I know it is not working?

19. ____ ____ Do I consider myself to be very competitive?

20. ____ ____ Do I not really trust myself or anyone else?

If you answered "yes" to three or more items, you need to do some healing in this regard. An exercise for reparenting yourself is presented in Chapter 6 as a tool you can use immediately.

For additional work in this area, you may also find the books listed in the Selected Bibliography very helpful, or you might want to access the services of a therapist specializing in this field. Patterns can be changed and cycles can be ended.

Common Problems of an Injured Inner Child

A wounded inner child may express many negative behaviors as a contaminated adult. Let us take a look at some of those behaviors that can impact your nursing career.

Codependency

Codependency is a state of confused identity resulting from the failure to move through the natural developmental stages of healthy dependence, independence, and interdependence. Being out of touch with your own feelings, desires, and needs and depending on externals for a definition of your identity are codependent responses. Making other people's problems your own is a common pattern because you are not clear about where you end and another person begins.

Many people who choose to go into the helping professions—nursing, social work, mental health, or the ministry—exhibit codependent behaviors. Because of the prevalence of this behavior pattern among nurses and its potential impact on your career, it will be explored in greater detail in Chapter 4.

Inappropriate Trusting

If a child grows up with parents who are not trustworthy, trust issues will arise when that child becomes an adult. The extremes of behavior range from controlling to giving up all control. Controllers feel safe and can trust only when all external events and people appear to be under their dominion. Others give up all control by gullibly overinvesting esteem in others. More subtle trust patterns also exist that fall somewhere between these two extremes. Those who have never learned to trust often have difficulty differentiating between control and security, obsession and caring, and intensity and intimacy. Lack of clarity in these areas can have a negative impact both on your nursing work and on your personal life.

Narcissism

If you did not feel loved unconditionally as a child, you may as an adult have a voracious internal demand for affection and attention. This can get played out in many ways. You may become a performer. Your stage need not be on Broadway. It may instead be on the job, where you act in a way that draws others around you in adulation. This star-like behavior serves as a mechanism that enables you to feel loved and appreciated.

Another common narcissistic behavior is addiction to ingestive substances such as alcohol, drugs, or food, where the substance serves as a substitute—albeit a poor one—for the love you desperately crave. An obsession with material possessions is still another narcissistic pattern, where you define yourself by what you own. The underlying thought is, "If I have all these things, I must be a wonderful person."

Narcissists can also become addicted to activity. As a nurse, you may find yourself volunteering for extra duties, taking on overtime, or providing unsolicited assistance to your colleagues. You are very busy and make yourself busier all the time. This, again, is another illusionary way of feeding yourself and, at the same time, distracting yourself from your authentic self.

Intimacy Confusion

The person without a concrete sense of self is bound to experience confusion about intimacy. Having a clear sense of identity about what is self and what is other is extremely important in nursing because so much of the daily interpersonal contact is intimate in nature. Your desire to be liked or to avoid hurting another's feelings may be at the root of behavior problems in this area.

The development of boundaries is essential for healthy functioning. It is important to set limits on the things you will do for others and what you will allow others to do to you. One way to create boundaries is to inform others of your position, make your behavior congruent with your verbiage, and hold others accountable for respecting your position. For example, in responding to a demanding patient whose needs are not immediate, rather than succumbing you may simply state, "I can't help you right now, but I can in 15 minutes."

Dysfunctional Family Roles

In a family that is not healthy, the children often adopt roles to get the attention they need. The authentic self of the little boy or girl becomes repressed and in its place arises, for example, the superachiever, the star, the rebel, the nice girl, or the caretaker. You may play multiple roles at one time or change roles as you grow. You may, for instance, be a rebel at ten and a superachiever at 15.

Early childhood stages provide the foundation for adulthood. If the foundation is not solid, the adult may get caught in behavior patterns that are not really productive for the growth and nurturance of a balanced and healthy person. The enacted roles of the child may become the adult's modus operandi. If, for example, you felt loved as a child only when you felt needed, you might adopt the caretaker role. This behavior allowed you to survive your family situation, but as an adult pattern, particularly for a nurse, it can make you very vulnerable to unhealthy codependency behaviors and contribute to professional burnout.

ADULT TRAUMAS

Just as most of us have experienced less than perfect childhoods, most of us have had some experiences as adults that may have been difficult or traumatizing. You may have gone through a tumultuous divorce or be currently involved in an unhappy marriage. You may be unable to get over the loss of a loved one. You may have physical challenges that have changed your life. Or you may currently be confused about your career direction. Everyone has been through disappointments and disillusionments and experienced uncertainty.

If you have not come to terms with such experiences, you are carrying emotional baggage. Like physical baggage, emotional baggage can slow you down, tire you out, and affect both your work performance and your personal happiness. Adult traumas, like childhood experiences, also need to be released. Chapter 6 provides you with ways of letting go and moving on.

SELECTED BIBLIOGRAPHY

Beattie, M., *Beyond Codependency and Getting Better All the Time.* New York: Harper & Row Publishers, Inc., 1989.

Beattie, M., *Codependent No More: How to Stop Controlling Others and Start Caring for Yourself.* New York: Harper & Row Publishers, Inc., 1987.

Bloomfield, H. and Felder, L. *Making Peace with Your Parents: The Key to Enriching Your Life and All Your Relationships.* New York: Ballantine, 1983.

Borysenko, J. *Minding the Body, Mending the Mind.* New York: Bantam Books, 1987.

Bradshaw J. *Homecoming: Reclaiming and Championing Your Inner Child.* New York: Bantam Books, 1990.

Buckley, C. D. and Walker, D. *Harmony: Professional Renewal for Nurses.* Chicago: American Hospital Publishing, Inc., 1989.

Capacchione, L. *Recovery of Your Inner Child.* New York: Simon & Schuster, 1991.

Hamilton, J. M. and Kiefer, M. E. *Survival Skills for Nurses.* Philadelphia: J. B. Lippincott Co., 1986.

Hay, L. L. *You Can Heal Your Life.* Santa Monica: Hay House, 1987.

Muller, W. *Legacy of the Heart: The Spiritual Advantages of a Painful Childhood.* New York: Simon & Schuster, 1992.

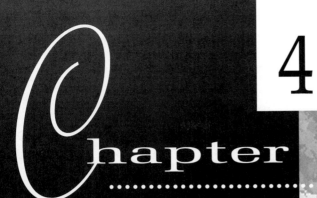

Chapter 4

From
Codependency
to
Interdependency

CODEPENDENCY CHARACTERISTICS

Codependency is a behavior pattern characterized by loss of identity. Individuals expressing this pattern do not have a realistic sense about who they are in relation to themselves or others. As a result they experience confusion about other people's needs and their own. The healthy boundary between *me* and *them* either does not exist, or if it does, it is full of holes.

As we mentioned in Chapter 3, codependency is very common in the helping professions. Most individuals expressing codependent behaviors tend to have been raised in dysfunctional families, where normal, healthy development is hindered. In dysfunctional families there is usually a prohibition on direct, honest communication and the expression of true feelings. This type of repression deprives children of the means to discover their true natures and learn appropriate responses to others.

CODEPENDENT BEHAVIOR PATTERNS

The two types of codependent behavior patterns are: narcissistic and caretaking. The *narcissistic* pattern operates from the perspective "You are responsible for how I feel." The individual expressing narcissistic behavior requires constant attention from others and feels angry or neglected when others do not cater to her desires. The *caretaking* pattern, on the other end of the fulcrum, operates in the mode "I am responsible for how you feel."

Individuals exhibiting the caretaking pattern often grow up in families that force them to assume caretaking activities at an early age in order to survive. Common scenarios are families with an alcoholic parent, or with a mother who has severe emotional problems and suffers from periodic breakdowns, or with an irresponsible father and a mother who must work. Any of these scenarios requires the family's young children to assume far greater responsibilities than they are prepared for emotionally. When young children grow up taking care of others, they often do not learn how to value or care for themselves.

EXPRESSING CODEPENDENCY AS A NURSE

Caretaking

Nurses who express codependent behaviors tend most often to exhibit the caretaking rather than the narcissistic pattern. Caretaking behavior puts others' needs before your own, often to the extent of neglecting or even harming yourself.

If you are expressing caretaking codependency, you are likely to let other people's behavior affect you more than it should and to feel far more responsible for others than is realistic. In other words, you tend to react rather than act, to be an effect rather than a cause.

As a nurse, you are a professional paid to take care of needy people. Your job requires you to provide for patients what they cannot provide for themselves. Some patients may respond quickly to your plan of care, while others may be demanding and uncooperative, and challenge your energy and creativity. People who are ill are often frightened, feel out of control, and lack the coping tools to adapt to a life-threatening situation.

Assisting patients, and sometimes their families and friends, to achieve a reasonable level of wellness can often be challenging and draining. Thus you can see why it is so important to have clear boundaries between you and your patients. It is also important to establish boundaries with your coworkers, family, and friends as the behavior pattern you express is not limited to your interactions with patients.

Rescuing Others

If you are acting codepenently, your parents probably did not value you appropriately when you were growing up. Thus as an adult you do not feel good about yourself. Having low self-esteem, you do not feel lovable. Instead, you settle for being needed because rescuing others makes you feel valued. It is easy for you to take on others' responsibilities while ignoring your own needs.

In rescuing others whom you view as victims, you become a victim yourself. By repeatedly rescuing others, you put yourself in a cycle of giving more than you receive. Reacting to this drain on your energies, you become angry and resentful because you are doing things you really do not want to do. Then you feel guilty about being resentful, often because your inculcated religious belief you are your brothers' keeper is paramount. All the while you consistently forget or overlook the other fundamental religious charges to love yourself as you love your neighbor and to care for your body as a temple.

Feeling neglected and used, you may end up feeling victimized. Like the north and south poles of magnets, your willingness to be a victim attracts perpetrators, and the cycle continues on.

Identifying Your Codependent Tendencies

Codependency plays out in a variety of ways. The questionnaire in Figure 4-1 lists a variety of feelings, thoughts, and actions that reflect codependency. Answer "yes" or "no" to each question, reflecting on both the professional and personal aspects of your life. Being honest with yourself may be difficult, but avoiding the truth may be harmful to your well-being.

FIGURE 4-1
Caretaking Codependent Behavior Questionnaire

	Yes	No	
1.			Do I feel responsible for other people's well-being and destiny?
2.			Do I feel compelled to help people solve their problems, even if they do not ask for my assistance?
3.			Do I usually end up doing more than my fair share of a group project?
4.			Do I do things for other people that they are capable of doing for themselves?
5.			Do I feel that I do not know what I really want or need?
6.			Do I feel safest when giving?
7.			Do I find it easier to talk about injustices others experience than about injustices I experience?
8.			Do I feel guilty, undeserving, or insecure when people give to me?
9.			Am I attracted to needy people, and are needy people attracted to me?
10.			Do I feel bored and empty if I do not have someone to help?
11.			Do I feel unappreciated, used, or angry?
12.			Do I come from a dysfunctional family, even though I do not like to admit it to myself or others?

	Yes	No	

13. ____ ____ Am I never satisfied with how I look, feel, behave, or think?

14. ____ ____ Do I feel guilty about spending money on myself or doing fun things?

15. ____ ____ Do I feel a lot of guilt?

16. ____ ____ Do I feel ashamed of who I am or feel that I am not quite good enough?

17. ____ ____ Have I been a victim of sexual, physical or emotional abuse, abandonment, or neglect?

18. ____ ____ Do I feel I need to be needed?

19. ____ ____ Do I get good feelings about myself from helping others, particularly in a crisis?

20. ____ ____ Do I think and talk a lot about other people and their problems?

21. ____ ____ Do I try to control events and people through manipulation, domination, or guilt?

22. ____ ____ Do I ignore problems or pretend they are not happening?

23. ____ ____ Do I overcommit myself to activities so I do not have to think about what is really going on?

24. ____ ____ Do I look for things and people to make me happy?

25. ____ ____ Do I feel I need people more than I want them?

26. ____ ____ Do I routinely seek love from people who are not capable of loving?

27. ____ ____ Do I not take time to see if other people are good for me before getting involved with them?

28. ____ ____ Do I not take myself seriously?

29. ____ ____ Do I routinely not say what I mean or mean what I say?

30. ____ ____ Do I have trouble saying "no" when someone asks for my help, even if it will create hardship for me?

31. ____ ____ Do I avoid talking about myself, particularly my feelings?

32. ____ ____ Do I have trouble expressing my emotions openly and honestly?

33. ____ ____ Do I feel other people's needs are more important than mine?

34. ____ ____ Do I let others hurt me and continue to hurt me?

35. ____ ____ Do I not trust myself?

36. ____ ____ Do I tend to trust untrustworthy people?

37. ____ ____ Do I feel scared, hurt, and angry deep inside?

38. ____ ____ Do I often cry or get depressed?

39. ____ ____ Do I act hostile, say nasty things to get even, or have violent temper tantrums?

	Yes	No	
40.	___	___	Do I feel ashamed when I get angry?
41.	___	___	Do I overeat, drink alcohol, or take drugs when I am angry?
42.	___	___	Do I have difficulty feeling close to people?
43.	___	___	Do I have trouble having fun and being spontaneous?
44.	___	___	Do I sacrifice my happiness for causes that do not require sacrifice?
45.	___	___	Do I stay loyal to people even if I continue being hurt?

The purpose of the exercise in Figure 4-1 is to identify individual behaviors, thoughts, or feelings that are problems for you and to become aware of your overall pattern of relating to others. Do not judge the behaviors or label yourself. This is not a situation involving "wrong" or "bad" behavior.

What you are looking for are indications of a state of imbalance that can create both emotional and physical stress for you, potentially leading to disease or burnout. Acknowledging that less than healthy behaviors exist is the first step toward setting positive change in motion.

ADDRESSING CODEPENDENT BEHAVIORS

With your new awareness and acceptance of any codependent behaviors that you may currently be expressing, you are now ready to take some actions to create healthful changes for yourself.

Looking at and Completing Your Unfinished Childhood Business

Looking at your childhood means being honest with yourself, about what your childhood was really like, even though this can be very painful. It is difficult to admit to yourself that mom and dad were not healthy and that, even though they did the best they knew how to do, they did not parent you well.

After looking at and accepting the reality of your upbringing, the next step is to engage in activities that heal the wounds of your childhood. Chapter 6 will provide you with some tools for accomplishing this.

Creating Boundaries

Figuring out where you end and someone else begins is crucial for a nurse. If your definition of your boundaries is not clear, you open yourself up to being drained by the people for whom you are caring as well as by your coworkers, family, and friends. Knowing what feelings are yours and which are someone else's is part of the process of defining boundaries. This may sound obvious, but for people who never were given the opportunity to know themselves, it may be quite difficult.

As you look at your childhood and become aware that you really do not have a good sense of your boundaries, some of the feelings you may experience are grief, sadness, and anger. It is important that you feel your feelings. Once you feel them and know that they belong to you and no one else, release them and let them go. Consult Chapter 6 for more help in this area.

Once you move past the expression, acceptance, and release of your feelings, you may find it useful to make a list of your likes and dislikes using the table in Figure 4-2. If you have been operating codependently, you may find that your initial list contains many items that are not really your own likes and dislikes but those of others to whom you have been close. If this is your experience, generate a second list, really tuning into what you, and only you, like and dislike. This exercise is very helpful in clarifying your borders.

Learning to Depend on Yourself for Your Happiness

Rather than depending on externals for your happiness, look within yourself. Grasping at unhealthy relationships or acquiring material things will not bring you lasting contentment. Externals change. If you can develop a strong sense of self-love and learn to care for yourself, you have within you an eternal source of happiness.

MOVING FROM CODEPENDENCY TO INERDEPENDENCY

The natural stages of healthy human development involve moving from a state of dependency to a state of independence and, ultimately, to a state of interdependency.

FIGURE 4-2
Personal Likes and Dislikes

Likes	Dislikes

If you are in a state of dependency or codependency, you need others to define who you are and to satisfy your needs. You are other-empowered rather than self-empowered. You are dependent on your environment, allowing the actions of others to determine your reactions.

Being independent requires that you be proactive—that you, and only you, choose how you respond to your environment. Being proactive requires that you respect and value yourself, develop self-confidence, and rely on your inner wisdom to make life-affirming choices. Being proactive and independent means that you take the initiative, are assertive, and make and keep commitments.

In healing your childhood wounds, establishing clear boundaries, and learning to love and nurture yourself you are in essence learning how to be independent. Only when you are independent can you become interdependent.

Being interdependent allows you to engage in the synergy of true sharing without losing your individual identity and independence. Interdependency is a bountiful state of being in which the fruits of the interaction are always richer and more plentiful than those produced individually.

SELECTED BIBLIOGRAPHY

Beattie, M. *Beyond Codependency and Getting Better All the Time.* New York: Harper & Row, 1989.

Beattie, M. *Codependent No More: How to Stop Controlling Others and Start Caring for Yourself.* New York: Harper & Row, 1987.

Briles, J. *The Confidence Factor.* New York: Master Media Limited, 1990.

Chenevert, M. *STAT: Special Techniques in Assertiveness Training,* 2nd ed. St. Louis: C. V. Mosby, 1983.

Covey, S. R. *The 7 Habits of Highly Effective People.* New York: Simon & Schuster, 1990.

Melody, P., Miller, A. W., and Miller, J. K. *Facing Codependence.* San Francisco: Harper & Row, 1989.

Melody, P. and Miller, A. W. *Breaking Free: A Recovery Workbook for Facing Codependence.* San Francisco: Harper & Row, 1989.

Schaef, A. W. *Co-Dependence: Misunderstood—Mistreated.* San Francisco: Harper & Row, 1986.

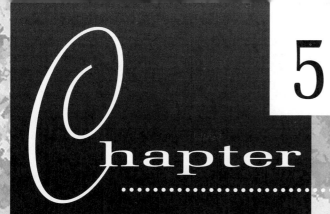

Chapter 5

From
Burnout to
Healthy
Helping

BURNOUT SYMPTOMS

Burnout was first described by psychoanalyst Herbert Feudenberger, who observed symptoms of physical, mental, and emotional exhaustion among clinic staff workers. Burnout occurs in all the helping professions and is quite common among nurses. It is a chronic condition manifesting a range of symptoms from physical problems, weariness, depression, anger, and hostility to withdrawal.

Escalating and continual emotional overload is a common factor in burnout. As a nurse you are under emotional stress daily as you deal with patients' problems, the demands of your coworkers and superiors, and the limits of the bureaucratic system in which you work. Support and positive feedback are often limited or nonexistent.

Although individual tolerance varies, the body eventually reacts to this prolonged stress arousal, reaching a point where extreme exhaustion sets in and symptoms of burnout begin to occur. You may find yourself moving from a position of being positive and caring to one of being negative and uncaring. You may become irritable, short-tempered, impatient, or withdrawn. You may find yourself overeating, imbibing alcohol, or ingesting drugs in increasing amounts. We are not talking here about "having a bad day." That happens to everyone. Rather, we are talking about a shift in your behavior that is chronic.

BURNOUT DEMOGRAPHICS

Men and women experience about the same incidence of burnout but tend to express it in different ways. Women become more emotionally exhausted, while men become depersonalized, detaching themselves from the people for whom they are caring. Burnout occurs more frequently in younger than in older workers, and the two-year mark on the job following training seems to be a critical point. Singles experience burnout more often than marrieds, and marrieds with children have less burnout than those without children.

LOSS OF IDEALISM

One cause of burnout is the gap between idealism and realism. Nursing school, like other schools for helping professionals, nurtures idealism. However, many who teach have not been on the front lines for years. Their memories may be vague about the daily challenges of nursing, or they may not be aware of the current demands on a staff nurse. Additionally, faculty are often constrained from presenting the "reality" of the institutional world by their dependence on these same institutions for student placements.

The pictures painted in school and the day-to-day realities of nursing can differ enormously. This gap between the culture of nursing school and the daily demands of working in the hospital was labeled "reality shock" by Dr. Marlene Kramer, author of a pioneering study of the same name.

Some realities of the work world include facing an unclear concept of what a nurse is, dealing with the attitudes of older physicians who may still consider nurses to be handmaidens, and needing to be constantly "up" and "on." Loss of idealism as a source of burnout is reflected in the demographics of nurses leaving the profession. The highest incidence of withdrawal is among young professionals after two years on the job. Weaving the cultures of school and work together into a third reality may be too demanding for young nurses, who may not yet have achieved the maturity required for this task.

Depression is a common symptom among nurses whose burnout is related to loss of idealism, since this experience involves letting go of a false belief. Loss feelings of mourning, grief, and sadness are typical.

CHARACTERISTICS OF THE BURNOUT-PRONE NURSE

Certain personality and behavioral characteristics increase the probability of experiencing burnout. As many of these traits are expressions of codependency, you can see the importance of healing codependent patterns before they lead you into burnout.

Self-Concept

Caregivers with low self-esteem and limited confidence are more prone to burnout than are those with more positive self-concepts. If you do not have a sense of self-worth, you seek assurance from others of your worthiness. Depending on others for self-validation can be emotionally dangerous, since the external validation you feel you need may not be consistently forthcoming from your patients or coworkers.

In the face of low self-esteem, when things are not going as you wish, they become obstacles rather than challenges. You tend to feel vulnerable and powerless, and your world view tends toward "the glass is half-empty" rather than "the glass is half-full." Your modus operandi is reactive rather than proactive. Over time this type of attitude is very depleting.

Limit Setting

A realistic appraisal of your unique strengths and weaknesses is important in establishing realistic limits for yourself. Admitting to yourself that certain areas of life are not particularly easy for you is not a sign of weakness. The danger of not admitting your limits is that you can easily overextend yourself.

Nurses, like other helping professionals, all too often fall into the "Messiah Trap," carrying false beliefs such as "It will not get done unless I do it," "I am the only one capable of doing it" or "It is my responsibility to save everyone." Acknowledging your humanness, your state of being less than perfect, is important preventive medicine for avoiding burnout.

Personal Needs

Although intellectual challenge and altruism are common motivating factors for selecting nursing as a career, personal needs may also enter into the decision.

Some caregivers have strong needs for approval and affection. Others may have difficulty in establishing close personal relationships and look to their work to satisfy their intimacy needs. Still others use nursing to boost their self-esteem. Guilt too, is sometimes a personal motivator, since nursing may seem to provide a suitable environment for expiating guilt through good deeds.

Some caregivers view nursing not just as a job but as an expression of personal identity, a personal mission. Others select a career in helping others as a way to avoid focusing on their own problems.

Relying on your career for satisfying personal needs such as intimacy, affection, approval, or identity can put you at great risk for burnout. Nursing involves giving and serving others. It does provide positive strokes that may satisfy some of your personal needs, and that is wonderful. The trick is not to expect your career to satisfy your deep personal needs. It is not the responsibility of your career to do that. It is your responsibility to create ways to satisfy your personal needs in the context of your personal life.

Fear

Nurses who have difficulty confronting their fears are more vulnerable to burnout than those who face their fears. Fear of death and personal loss is something that as a nurse you must address because these realities are a part of your daily environment. Avoiding or denying fear can lead to psychic numbing, or cutting yourself off from all your feelings.

Coming to terms with your fears is the only way to deal with them. First, acknowledge your fears and accept them as legitimate expressions of your feelings. Then make friends with your fears. Learning to grieve and to let go is an important survival tool. Supportive colleagues who experience the same daily environment you do and have mastered their fears can be very helpful in assisting you to work through yours.

Empathy

A direct relationship exists between emotional empathy and burnout. The ability to feel another person's pain as your own increases your susceptibility to emotional exhaustion. Setting boundaries and knowing what is your patient's pain and what is your pain is essential for preventing burnout. Cognitive or detached empathy is a healthier position to take. You are aware of your patient's pain and have compassion for it, but you do not experience it. This realization is a shift in view from "their pain is my pain" to "their pain is their pain."

Attachment to Results

Nurses who are attached to seeing positive results as a direct reflection of their efforts are also vulnerable to burnout. Sometimes, no matter what you do or how hard you work, the result is not what you want it to be. Attachment to results breeds frustration, and prolonged frustration leads to exhaustion.

One way to reframe how you view results is to look at success as a combination of results, processes, and relationships. Know that you made a difference in your patients' care by being there for them, not only as a caretaker but as a companion on their journey to wellness.

ENVIRONMENTAL FACTORS IN BURNOUT

Additional factors contribute to burnout other than personality and behavioral characteristics. These factors are environmental and are directly related to the nature of the nursing work setting.

Burnout is high when you feel you do not have control over the quality of care you are delivering. Institutional rules, supervisor rigidity, coworker attitudes, or budgetary restrictions may contribute to your feelings of frustration.

Support Groups

Establishing a support group among your professional colleagues may be helpful. Sharing with others experiencing the same stresses can relieve your sense of isolation, provide emotional support, and be a source of positive feedback.

Precautions must be taken, however, to ensure that the group does not succumb to confrontations or chronic complaining. The group should be structured in such a way that each member is encouraged to speak up and to make an effort to understand the others, more seasoned members serve as mentors or counselors, and a clearly defined process exists for group decision making.

Making Choices

It is your challenge to change what you can to make the environment more conducive to your productivity and well-being. However, it is also important to realize that institutional change is very slow, and that some factors such as budgetary constraints may not be affected by your efforts.

If you find that conditions remain static, you have two choices. You can change your way of dealing with the environment. By adopting a proactive approach, you can choose to respond in new, more constructive ways to the same stimuli. Or you may decide that the only feasible solution for you is to change positions within your institution or to seek employment elsewhere.

WARNING SIGNS OF BURNOUT

The best way to prevent burnout is early detection of symptoms. Pay attention to the comments of your colleagues, friends, and relatives.

They may prove to be your best early warning system by noticing negative changes in you before you do.

It is also a good idea to take a look at yourself periodically. Figure 5-1 is a self-assessment tool for burnout. Answering these questions every three to six months, particularly if you are remaining in the same work environment, can provide you with a valuable reflection of attitudes and behaviors that may be precursors or indicators of burnout. Acknowledging any of the symptoms listed should serve as an alert to you about your potential for burnout.

FIGURE 5-1
Burnout Questionnaire

During the last three __ six __ months I have been:

1. ___ Having headaches on a regular basis
2. ___ Having chronic backaches
3. ___ Having nightmares regularly
4. ___ Having difficulty sleeping
5. ___ Sleeping more than usual
6. ___ Depressed
7. ___ Irritable
8. ___ Using alcohol and drugs to escape
9. ___ Spending more and more time alone
10. ___ Feeling angry or hostile
11. ___ Feeling numb and disinterested in everything
12. ___ Feeling emotionally drained
13. ___ Feeling as though I am not accomplishing anything on my job
14. ___ Disinterested in my patients' welfare
15. ___ Hating going to work
16. ___ Taking long breaks and lunches
17. ___ Feeling dissatisfied with everything in my life

ADDRESSING BURNOUT

If you see that you are walking down the path to burnout, there are some actions you should take immediately.

Set Realistic Goals for Yourself

Instead of remaining immersed in the notion of "saving all the sick and needy in the world," develop some realistic goals for yourself that will provide you with a sense of accomplishment. "Attending to the needs of my patients to the best of my abilities and within the constraints of the institutional setting" is a realistic goal. "Having a positive and caring attitude toward my patients" is another achievable goal.

After you receive your assignment and before you start your shift, establish reasonable expectations for yourself, your team, and your patients for that day. Acknowledge your successes and reward yourself when something goes well.

Create and Enjoy Your Breaks

Take your breaks, particularly if your tendency is to feel you cannot afford the time to take them. Get away from your patients and do something enjoyable. Sometimes just going off by yourself is a healing relief from the intense interaction of your work.

Take Care of Yourself

Make sure that you create time in your life for rest and relaxation. Do things you enjoy—sports, hobbies, art, music, being with friends and loved ones. It is essential to create a personal life that nurtures you and balances the demands of your professional life.

Healthy Helping

Nursing Is One Part of the Whole

Nursing is not your life. You are not your job. You are not your career. Nursing is one of many things you do in your life. It can bring you much satisfaction or it can drain you. The choice is yours. Know where nursing belongs in the larger context of your complete life.

You Are Here to Serve, Not to Rescue

Looking at yourself as someone who is providing a service is much healthier than seeing yourself as a rescuer. Rescuers maintain victims and become victims themselves. Do not get caught in the "Messiah Trap." Know your strengths, recognize areas with room for growth, and establish clear boundaries. Do the best job you are capable of doing, but do not get attached to the results of your efforts. Some patients get sicker or die, regardless of your ministrations.

Find a Comfortable Place for Yourself

Some nurses thrive in emergency care, intensive care, or surgery. Others do not do well in these settings. Find the right place for your talents. Nursing offers a variety of opportunities. Find those that fit you. Do not try to be a round peg in a square hole.

Learn Appropriate Empathy

Understanding someone's pain on a cognitive level is healthier than feeling that person's pain. A certain level of detachment is necessary for effective caregiving and self-preservation. Establishing your boundaries is an important step in this process.

Create Support for Yourself

Establish solid relationships with friends and supportive colleagues who can really be there for you. Because you are giving so much, you need to make sure that you are receiving as well. Do not discount the importance of this support. Make time in your life to develop these relationships, both personally and professionally.

Heal Your Own Wounds

A wounded healer is not an effective healer. Working on your own unhealthy patterns is the greatest gift you can give to yourself and to your patients.

Love Yourself

Loving yourself is sometimes easier said than done for caregivers, who are conditioned to giving all the time. You need to give to yourself in order to continue to be able to give to others. Self-love can take many forms. Do things you enjoy because you enjoy them. Buy yourself something because you like it. Treat yourself the way you wish ideally to treat your patients, with optimism, sincerity, consideration, and attentiveness. Loving yourself well allows you to care for others in a loving way.

SELECTED BIBLIOGRAPHY

Alberti, R. E. and Emmons, M. *Your Perfect Right: A Guide to Assertive Living,* 5th rev. ed. San Luis Obispo: Impact Publishers, 1986.

Briles, J. *The Confidence Factor: How Self-Esteem Can Change Your Life.* New York: Master Media Limited, 1990.

Covey, S. *The 7 Habits of Highly Effective People.* New York: Simon & Schuster, 1990.

Kramer, M. *Reality Shock: Why Nurses Leave Nursing.* St. Louis: C. V. Mosby, 1974.

Kramer, M. and Schmalenberg, C. *Path to Biculturalism.* Wakefield, MA: Contemporary Publishing, 1977.

Luks, A. and Payne, P. *The Healing Power of Doing Good: The Health and Spiritual Benefits of Helping Others.* New York: Ballantine Books, 1991.

Maslach, C. *Burnout: The Cost of Caring.* Englewood Cliffs, NJ: Prentice-Hall, 1982.

Chapter 6

Mindcise: Exercises for the Mind

THE MIND

The function of the mind is to think. It is through thought that you define yourself, your environment, and your place in the world. Whether conscious or unconscious, present or past, your thoughts impact every facet of your life.

DEFINING AND RESEARCHING THE MIND

Psychoneuroimmunology research has scientifically demonstrated the impact of thoughts and feelings on the body. Positive thoughts and feelings are now known to be health-promoting, while negative thoughts and feelings are stress-producing.

Recent research at Stanford University and the University of California, Berkeley, conducted by psychologists Felicia Pratto and Oliver John, presents some interesting revelations regarding unconscious perception and the memory of positive and negative thoughts (*Newsweek,* Note 1).

Study volunteers viewed a series of typed words flashed onto a computer screen in a variety of colors. Common words were used, including negatives such as "dishonest" or "miserly" and their opposite positive qualities. When asked to name the colors in which the words were displayed, respondents took longer to name the colors of negative words, suggesting that their attention focused longer on the words themselves than on the attribute of color. The study participants also recalled more negative words than positive ones.

THE CHOICE IS YOURS

If we as humans tend unconsciously to remember and perceive more negatives than positives, it may be because our culture immerses us in that sort of climate. For example, how much of the news reported in the media is positive? Occasionally, there is an inspirational "human interest" story in the midst of all the reports on chaos, corruption, destruction, and deception. But the predominant message is negative.

As a nurse you are occupationally trained to look for the negative—what is wrong, what is abnormal, and so forth. This viewpoint, of course, is necessary if you are to assist your patients, but it also constitutes another subtle imprinting that becomes part of your internal thought environment.

The mind, however, makes a choice about how it thinks. As Shakespeare's Hamlet noted, "There is nothing good nor bad but thinking that makes it so." Regardless of what is going on in your world, you choose a positive or negative thinking mode, consciously or unconsciously. And you can choose consciously to shift from the negative to the positive.

The choice you make is important because how you view the world is how it gets reflected back to you. For example, the owner of a small urban business complained continually about how run-down the city had become, what undesirable characteristics certain ethnic groups had, and how terrible the economy was. Then his business was robbed. He saw no relation between the negativity of his thoughts and the corresponding negative event he had just experienced. On the other end of the spectrum are people like Helen Keller, who despite severe physical handicaps lived a full, productive, and inspirational life with the attitude: "One cannot consent to creep when one feels the impulse to soar!"

Your world is as your mind sees it. Your thoughts draw the experiences associated with those thoughts to you. If, for example, you believe the world is harmful, you will be harmed. If, on the other hand, you believe the world is full of infinite possibilities, that is what you will experience.

ATTITUDES AND BELIEFS

Attitudes and beliefs are the foundation underlying our thoughts. Some attitudes and beliefs are conscious, while others may be more elusive. The sources of attitudes and beliefs are multiple, including childhood upbringing, societal imprinting, and environmental experiences.

It is important to focus in consciously on your beliefs and attitudes and to identify any that are no longer helping you to attain what you want and be who you want to be. By looking at attitudes and beliefs, you can identify areas from your past that are withholding part of your energy from you in the present. Any area of your inner life that is stuck in the past takes energy away from you. Stored negative memories, in essence, may be preventing you from experiencing a fuller, more joyful life.

Spend some time listing your current adult attitudes, using Figure 6-1. List at least two attitudes for each category. If this comes slowly or is difficult for you, you may find it useful to set the questionnaire aside for a few days and then come back to it.

You may want to refer back to the questionnaires on the injured child in Chapter 3 and codependency in Chapter 4 for help in completing the childhood beliefs section of the chart. An example of a childhood belief that may still be functioning as an adult attitude is: "I am lazy." If your mother repeatedly said those words to you when you did not want to clean up your room at her request, that belief may still be affecting your self-concept as an adult.

After you complete all categories in Figure 6-1, take a look at the relationship between your childhood beliefs and your adult attitudes.

THE POWER OF WORDS

Words express thoughts and are thus very powerful. It is important to choose your words carefully because you can use them to change negative situations or conditions to positive ones. For example, saying: "I am a codependent" is very different from saying: "I am acting codependently" or "I am experiencing codependent behaviors." If you are "acting" or "experiencing," you are engaged in a temporary behavior. You have experienced many things and acted in many ways in the past, and you will experience many other things and act in many other ways in the future if you choose to do so.

However, if you say: "I am a codependent" or "I am fat" or "I am an alcoholic," you are claiming that position as your identity and fixing it there. The words "I am" can just as readily be used positively to establish a new identity, a new position for yourself. Saying: "I am fat" will keep you fat. Saying: "I am thin and energetic," on the other hand, will help move you into that new position.

Words create a mental atmosphere. Begin watching your own language and that of others. For example, a friend may call you on a regular

FIGURE 6-1
Beliefs and Attitudes

1. Current attitudes about career

_____
_____
_____
_____
_____
_____

2. Current attitudes about relationships

_____
_____
_____
_____
_____
_____

3. Current attitudes about body and health

_____
_____
_____
_____
_____
_____

4. Current attitudes about money

_____
_____
_____
_____
_____
_____

5. Childhood beliefs that may still be functioning as adult attitudes

_____
_____
_____
_____
_____

basis and say: "Well, let's see, the crisis of the week was..." Or you may know a man who always says: "Business is great," even when he has not seen a customer for days. Watch the language of your colleagues, friends, and relatives. Notice which ones get sick more often or have minor catastrophes all the time, and match what they are experiencing with what they are saying.

AFFIRMATIONS

To affirm means to declare the existence of, assert to be true, state positively. Affirmations can thus be a tool for changing a negative to a positive. In a sense, using affirmations is like reprogramming a computer. The new program is inserted over the old, replacing the old beliefs with new ones. Affirmations are not a new idea. Affirmative prayer has been used for centuries by various religious disciplines.

The first step in using an affirmation to change a condition is to identify the belief(s) or attitude(s) associated with the condition. For example, you may have the attitude that you will always be overweight because you believe being overweight is a family trait. By clinging to: "I will always be overweight," you are, in essence, stating that you are overweight now and that this condition will never change in the future.

To establish a new reality for yourself in the present, change the belief to "I am thin and energetic, and I love how my body looks." By changing your belief, you are reframing a negative into a positive. Attention goes to where thought is. By focusing on the new positive image you make the old one fade and disappear. You could say it withers away and dies from lack of attention.

Affirmations work by bringing the future into the present through the exercise of the mind. Once you identify the condition you want to change and the associated belief(s) or attitude(s), create a one-sentence affirmation that defines the new condition, as shown in the examples in Figure 6-2.

FIGURE 6-2
Affirmation Examples

CONDITION	OLD BELIEF/ATTITUDE	AFFIRMATION
I am being drained by the needs of others.	Others are more important than I am.	I am important, and my needs are just as important as anyone else's.
I have very low self-esteem.	My parents were right when they said I would never amount to anything.	I am a valuable and worthwhile person deserving only the best.
My friends are not really there for me.	I need to have friends with problems so that I will feel needed.	I have friends who are there for me as much as I am there for them.
I am afraid to apply for a more responsible position.	I am not really capable.	I am capable of anything I undertake and excel in everything I do.

Repetition

Affirmations must be repeated to be effective. Repetition of the new idea replaces the old and establishes a new pattern. Once you have figured out an appropriate affirmation for your situation, write it down on note cards. Place the note cards where you will see them constantly, e.g.: on the refrigerator, on the mirrors, on closet doors. Carry one with you and use it often each day.

Begin by saying the affirmation aloud while standing in front of a mirror and looking yourself in the eyes. If your eyes tell you that you do not really believe what you are saying, ask yourself to reveal any additional beliefs and attitudes that are keeping you from doing so. Repeat this process until you believe what you are affirming.

If your environment permits, repeat your affirmation aloud. Otherwise, repeat it silently to yourself, closing your eyes and focusing all your attention on the thought. Feel it, really feel it, as you say it. The more real you can make it for yourself the more real it becomes for you. Repeat your affirmation at least 50 times a day.

Read the note card you carry with you when you are waiting in lines or at traffic lights. You may also want to make an audio tape of yourself repeating the affirmation and play that tape throughout the day and before you go to sleep.

To start with, work with just one affirmation at a time. As you become more comfortable with the process, you can add a few more. Continue with your affirming process until you feel the change in yourself and your environment begins reflecting the change back to you.

VISUALIZATION

Visualization is similar to affirmation in that it replaces a negative image with a positive one. Rather than being verbal, however, visualization is an exercise for the mind that uses pictures to create the new reality.

The effective use of visualization by athletes has been documented for years. Olympic and professional athletes often comment on their use of visualization to enhance their performance, and many books have been written on the inner games of tennis, skiing, and other sports. Scientific studies have recorded electrophysiological changes in the body due to simple visualization of the athletic activity. A combination of visual and kinesthetic imaging, during which the desired result is both seen and felt, has been found to be most effective in athletics.

Dr. Carl Simonton pioneered the medical use of visualization with cancer patients, and many other programs working with patients with degenerative diseases have adopted this approach. Visualization has also become a commonly employed tool of many top business executives.

A Sensory Experience

The key to successful visualization is to make it as real for yourself as you can. To do this, try to employ as many senses in the activity as you can. Paint a picture with your mind's eye, feel it, sense it, taste it, smell it, and hear it. Do not be concerned if you do not actually see the picture. It is enough to have a sense that it exists.

Jumping Back

Going back in your personal history and recreating that history is a very powerful tool for changing the present. Since so many people had less than ideal childhoods, that is the focus selected for the exercise presented here. This is, in essence, a reparenting experience. However, you may use this technique for any past experience, childhood or adult, that you want to recreate to change your present situation or condition.

Jumping Back: Reparenting

1. Sit or lie in a comfortable position with your eyes closed.

2. Go back to a childhood experience with your parents that was painful for you. Take whatever time you need to find that experience. It need not be the worst one, just one that you can still remember as a time when you felt that your parents did not support you.

3. Visualize all the people involved, what they look like, what they are wearing. See the room and notice the furnishings and the color of the walls. See as much detail as possible. Tune into the sounds, smells, temperature, tastes.

4. Reexperience the interactions that took place. Feel the pain, physical and/or emotional. Let yourself flow through the entire event.

5. Now release that picture and take a few deep breaths, completely clearing it from your consciousness. Forgive every one who did not act in the way you wanted, and forgive yourself for behaving in any way about which you did not feel right. The act of forgiving is the most important part of this exercise. Only by releasing the past can you truly move into a new present.

6. Create a new picture now about how you would have liked the experience to have been for you. Again, use all your senses and create as much detail as you did in the previous steps.

7. Experience the wonderful feelings of being loved, protected, honored, valued, and adored.

8. Remaining anchored in that experience, bring yourself back to a wakeful state.

Repeat this exercise until the new feelings become a part of you, until you really know that your inner child is loved, nurtured, supported, and healed.

Jumping Forward

Just as you can use visualization to recreate the past, you can use it to create the future in the present, just as you do with affirmations.

Jumping Forward: Creating the Ideal You

1. Sit or lie in a comfortable position with your eyes closed.

2. See yourself as you would like to be. Envision how you look, what you are wearing, what kind of work you are doing, your personal relationships, where you are living, what kind of car you are driving, and with whom you are living. Visualize yourself happy, healthy, and vibrant. Create the textures of your world, all the subtle nuances. Feel the feelings, smell the smells, hear the sounds, and taste the tastes. Really be there.

3. Hold this image in your mind until you are sure you can remember it. Then release it, take a few deep breaths, and return to wakeful consciousness.

Repeat this exercise as often as you like. You may want to keep a journal, recording the changes that occur in your life that match your pictures.

RIGHT AND LEFT TOGETHER

Think of affirmation and visualization as two parts which together comprise a whole. Affirmation uses the linear sequencing of language and is primarily a left-brain function. Visualization can be thought of as a round process, a nonverbal, pictorial activity, which is primarily a right-brain function. Another way to consider the combination of affirmation and visualization is to view them as complementary in nature, like the sun and the moon, or the Taoist yang and yin.

CREATING PRESENCE

As you reframe your outdated beliefs and attitudes, replacing them with new ones, you will bring more of yourself from the past into the present. Releasing those areas of your self that have been imprisoned in the past allows you to become a clearer, more focused, more energetic and positive person. The presence you create as you become more fully yourself is healing not only for you but for those around you—your patients, colleagues, family, and friends.

ON-SITE TOOLS

Up until this point we have looked at using mindcise tools to heal the past and to bring a better future into the present. These tools, however, can also be used in your daily work setting.

For example, suppose that you are experiencing communication difficulties with an authoritative physician. Rather than retreating to a placating position or engaging in confrontation, you can use visualization and affirmation to change how you experience the situation.

The Spiritual Perspective

From a spiritual perspective, visualize the physician as a whole, complete, and perfect being, and know that whatever behavior she is expressing is only behavior and not her true nature. An appropriate affirmation for this situation is: "Dr. Martin is whole, complete, and perfect, and any expression to the contrary is only temporary behavior, not her true nature."

The Humorous Perspective

From a humorous perspective, visualize the physician wearing nothing but a diaper standing in the middle of an exclusive department store. More than one prominent speaker has told stories of mitigating stage fright by such moments of humorous visualization.

NOTE

1. "What's so good about remembering the bad?" *Newsweek* (Nov. 2, 1992, p. 83.)

SELECTED BIBLIOGRAPHY

Fanning, P. *Visualization for Change.* Oakland: New Harbinger, 1988.

Hay, L. L. *A Garden of Thoughts: My Affirmation Journal.* Carson, CA: Hay House, 1989.

Hay, L. L. *The Power Is Within You.* Carson, CA: Hay House, 1991.

Holmes, E., and Kinnear, W. H. *A New Design For Living.* New York: Prentice Hall, 1987.

John-Roger, and McWilliams, P. *Life 101: Everything We Wish We Had Learned About Life In School—But Didn't.* Los Angeles: Prelude, 1991.

Matthews-Simonton, S., Simonton, O. C., and Creighton, J. L. *Getting Well Again.* New York: Bantam Books, 1987.

Ponder, C. *The Dynamic Laws of Healing.* 12th Ed. Marina del Rey: DeVorss, 1980.

Chapter 7

Meditation: Portable Peace

WHAT IS MEDITATION?

Meditation is a practice of all religious traditions, but you need not be religious to meditate or receive the benefits of meditation. Neither do you need a guru or meditation teacher, although many have benefitted from such assistance.

Whereas affirmation and visualization are active, meditation is receptive—the moon balancing the sun. Meditation is simply about being still, about quieting the mind and focusing it in the present, about releasing fears, worries, anxieties, and doubts concerning your yesterdays and tomorrows. Meditation is about being fully present in the here and now. It is not about making an effort. Rather it is about recognizing what is and letting it be—the peace, joy, harmony, and beauty that is you.

BENEFITS OF MEDITATION

Everyone needs to have a sense of belonging, of being connected. It is well documented that those who are isolated or feel isolated from others tend to have more health problems than those who do not experience such feelings. For example, when one spouse in a long-term marriage dies, it is not unusual for the remaining spouse, who may not have a strong social network, to get very ill or die within a short time. The feelings of separation and lack of harmony believed to account for this phenomenon are also common among—and equally detrimental to—both cancer and heart patients.

Meditation is a tool for knowing that you are part of something larger than yourself. That something is whatever is real for you: the human family, the universe, Spirit, nature, infinite energy, or God. Whatever it is for you does not matter. What does matter is the sense of connecting with something greater than your everyday world.

Research by Dr. Herbert Benson and others have shown that in comparison to nonmeditators, meditators are calmer, more focused, more productive, and less dependent on external events for their happiness. Other commonly reported benefits of meditation include increased feelings of harmony and oneness, a sense of well-being, enhanced energy and creativity, a lesser tendency to worry and be anxious, and lessened incidences of anger and hostility.

PHYSIOLOGICAL EFFECTS OF MEDITATION

Significant changes in the physiology of the body that occur during meditation have been researched by Dr. Robert Keith Wallace, Dr. Benson, and others (Wallace & Benson, Note 1). The metabolic rate, blood pressure, and oxygen consumption are lowered. The level of oxygen consumed during meditation is less than that consumed during either sleep or hypnosis. Meditation produces a state of deep rest combined with mental alertness (Wallace et al, Note 2).

Meditation also creates significant changes in cerebral cortical activity. In comparison to nonmeditators, meditators show increases in the slower, relaxing alpha and theta brainwaves. Increased synchronicity in the left and right brain hemispheres and in the front and back areas of the brain, with consistent uniformity in frequency and amplitude of the brainwaves, are additional findings. In ordinary waking consciousness there is no such synchronicity; the brainwaves are random and chaotic.

Other physiological research shows that blood lactate levels, associated with states of anxiety and tension, are far lower during meditation than during periods of quiet rest (Wallace et al, Note 3). Dr. David Orme-Johnson, measuring galvanic skin response, found that meditators have increased stability of the autonomic nervous system and improved adaptability and resistance to stress in comparison to nonmeditators (Orme-Johnson, Note 4).

Studies of the effects of meditative training on the immune system, performed by immunologist Dr. Ronald Glaser and psychologist Dr. Janice Kiecolt-Glaser, have shown increased NK- and T-cell activity as a result of the practice (Kiecolt-Glaser, Notes 5 and 6). Dr. Joan Borysenko reports a doubling in NK-cell activity in people who have a sense of connectedness relative to people who feel lonely and unconnected (Borysenko, Note 7). These findings coincide with the frequent self-reports of improved health in meditators.

PREPARING TO LEARN MEDITATION

Meditation involves two activities—relaxation and focused attention. If you have never meditated before, experience in these two areas can be quite helpful in preparing you for meditation practice.

Relaxation

Experiencing relaxation kinesthetically will assist you to know how your body should feel when you are meditating.

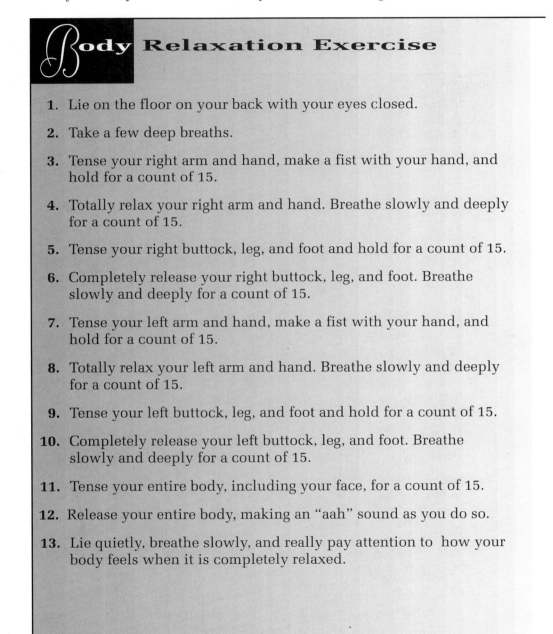

Body Relaxation Exercise

1. Lie on the floor on your back with your eyes closed.

2. Take a few deep breaths.

3. Tense your right arm and hand, make a fist with your hand, and hold for a count of 15.

4. Totally relax your right arm and hand. Breathe slowly and deeply for a count of 15.

5. Tense your right buttock, leg, and foot and hold for a count of 15.

6. Completely release your right buttock, leg, and foot. Breathe slowly and deeply for a count of 15.

7. Tense your left arm and hand, make a fist with your hand, and hold for a count of 15.

8. Totally relax your left arm and hand. Breathe slowly and deeply for a count of 15.

9. Tense your left buttock, leg, and foot and hold for a count of 15.

10. Completely release your left buttock, leg, and foot. Breathe slowly and deeply for a count of 15.

11. Tense your entire body, including your face, for a count of 15.

12. Release your entire body, making an "aah" sound as you do so.

13. Lie quietly, breathe slowly, and really pay attention to how your body feels when it is completely relaxed.

Concentration

Meditation is a relaxed state of mental alertness. One way to prepare yourself for the mental state of meditation is to perform a concentration exercise. Concentration means focusing your attention on one thing and one thing only.

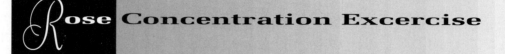

Rose Concentration Excercise

1. Buy or pick a rose that is not fully open.

2. Sit comfortably in a quiet space and close your eyes for a minute with the rose resting in one of your hands.

3. Open your eyes and look at the rose and nothing else.

4. Focus your attention first on one petal. Note the color, texture, shape, and size of the petal.

5. Now, move your attention from that petal to the adjacent one. Examine this petal with the same focused interest. Continue this process for each petal, noting how each petal is the same and yet different from the previous one.

6. After you have examined all of the petals, study each leaf on the stem, then move on to the stem itself, and finally to each thorn. Notice every small detail.

7. Now move the rose a short distance away from you and look at the rose in its completeness. Note its overall shape, form, color, and texture.

8. Smell the fragrance, taking a few slow, deep breaths. Then close your eyes and concentrate solely on the fragrance.

9. Open your eyes, look at the complete rose one more time, and inhale its fragrance.

10. Now, close your eyes and take the image of the rose into your heart. With your eyes closed, continue to smell the rose and see the rose in as much detail as you can with your mind's eye.

CREATING YOUR SPACE AND TIME FOR MEDITATION

It is important to establish a place to use consistently for meditation. This may be a certain chair, a particular section of a sofa, or a corner of a room with a cushion on the floor. What matters is that this is your dedicated meditation space. Make sure it is clean, orderly, quiet, and located in an area devoid of distractions. If there is a telephone nearby, turn off its sound during your meditation time.

You may put beautiful, uplifting, and inspirational objects in your meditation space if this idea appeals to you. For example, you may choose to place flowers, candles, incense, or anything you consider sacred or meaningful in your space.

Now that you have created a special place for meditation, you need also to select a special time during which you will meditate each day. If possible, select a time in the early morning or in the evening. Start with 5 minutes and gradually work up to 20-minute sessions once or twice a day. It is best not to eat for two hours before meditating so that your complete energy can be devoted to meditation rather than having part of that energy distracted by digestive demands.

By creating a special time and place for meditation, you are establishing a framework for a new and healthy habit. Give it attention and repeat it consistently, and meditation will serve you well.

POSITIONING YOUR BODY FOR MEDITATION

You may either sit cross-legged on the floor or upright in a straight-backed chair. Whatever position you choose, it is important that your spine be straight and your body relaxed. Do not meditate lying down as you will be prone to falling asleep. Wear comfortable, nonrestrictive clothing and make sure to loosen anything that may be binding around your waist.

WAYS TO MEDITATE

Concentration is the arrow and meditation the bow. Although there are many different meditation techniques or styles, all serve to bring peace, increase awareness, and clarify the mind.

You may choose among many ways to meditate—with structure, without structure, with eyes closed, with eyes open, sitting still, moving, and so on. No one way is better than any other. What is important is to find a way that fits you.

Although it is not possible to present all methods, two common methods for meditation are described below. One technique focuses on breathing, and the other focuses on a word or affirmative thought. You may want to explore both to discover which is more effective for you.

Focusing on Breathing

This style of meditation concentrates your attention on the flow of your breath.

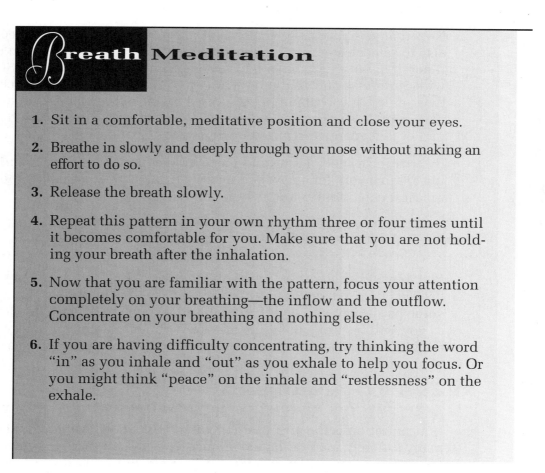

*B*reath Meditation

1. Sit in a comfortable, meditative position and close your eyes.

2. Breathe in slowly and deeply through your nose without making an effort to do so.

3. Release the breath slowly.

4. Repeat this pattern in your own rhythm three or four times until it becomes comfortable for you. Make sure that you are not holding your breath after the inhalation.

5. Now that you are familiar with the pattern, focus your attention completely on your breathing—the inflow and the outflow. Concentrate on your breathing and nothing else.

6. If you are having difficulty concentrating, try thinking the word "in" as you inhale and "out" as you exhale to help you focus. Or you might think "peace" on the inhale and "restlessness" on the exhale.

Focusing on a Word or Affirmative Thought

Another way to meditate is to concentrate on a word or affirmative thought. This method is known in Sanskrit as *mantra* meditation. Use of this technique was included as an optional step in the breathing meditation instructions, but it may also be used to good effect alone. Simply shift your attention away from breathing and toward the chosen word or phrase.

Select a word or phrase that helps you feel peaceful. The Sanskrit word *om* or *aum,* meaning "one" in English, is commonly used. Hindus believe that *om* is the universal sound, and that the vibrational quality of this sound assists in deepening meditation. Depending on your personal beliefs, you may want to select a spiritually significant word such as om, amen, shalom, one, or God. Or you may choose a secular word such as ocean, peace, or relax. You may either use a single word or expand that word to an affirmative phrase such as "I am at peace" or "I am one with God."

Interestingly, Dr. Benson found that when he offered his patients a choice of soothing words for mantra meditation, 80% selected a spiritually significant word or phrase. Those who chose a faith-related mantra remained with the program longer and showed greater improvement in health than did those who selected a secular word.

*M*antra Meditation

1. Sit in a comfortable, meditative position and close your eyes.

2. Select your word or phrase.

3. Establish a pattern of slow, steady, rhythmic breathing.

4. Repeat your word or phrase either aloud or silently on exhaling.

WATCHING YOUR THOUGHTS

One common experience most people have when they start to meditate is being distracted by their thoughts during their meditative practice. Hindus refer to this phenomenon as the activity of busy monkeys. As you quiet your mind you find out just how busy it really is.

It is best not to repress the thoughts as they appear, but simply watch them as they go by. Then bring your attention back to meditating—to your breathing or your mantra.

Some people find their minds filled with "to-do" lists as they begin to meditate and have great difficulty in letting go of these thoughts. If this is your experience, before you begin meditation, try concentrating on all the things you need to do that day, writing them down, and releasing them.

Do not be discouraged by the presence of thoughts during meditation. You are learning a new way of being with yourself. As with all new habits, it takes some time to acquire. Over time you will find that these intrusions lessen with practice.

WAYS TO GET DEEPER

Once you have mastered meditating for 20 minutes or more, you may find there are days when you have difficulty being as quiet as you would like to be. It may not be that thoughts are distracting you, but simply that you have a sense that you are not totally present in your meditation. The following tools may assist you to refocus.

Deep Breathing

Breathing deeply with an inhale, retention, and exhale ratio of 1:4:2 is a good way to center yourself and enter into a deeper meditative space. For detailed instruction on this technique, see Chapter 8.

Music

Audio tapes and CDs are available that have been designed specifically for meditation and have a calming, relaxing, and enhancing effect. Harp and flute pieces, Gregorian chants, and sounds of nature are examples of this type of music, usually categorized as relaxation or "New Age" in music stores. Elevating classical music by composers such as Pachelbel, Teleman, and Vivaldi are also good selections. Playing such music as you meditate may assist you in moving deeper in your practice.

Twirling

Twirl your body clockwise with your arms extended, as you did when you were a child, 21 times. When you stop twirling, sit in a meditative posture and close your eyes.

Group Meditation

There is power in a group of minds all focused in a meditative state. The synergy of the whole is far greater than the sum of the individuals. Many people find it useful to access this energy by meditating with others as a way of deepening their practice.

Sacred Places

In places where people have prayed or meditated for a number of years, the environment has become saturated with a calm, peaceful feeling. Sitting in a church, temple, hospital chapel, or other place of worship or spiritual ritual can assist you in entering into a deeper level of meditation.

PORTABLE PEACE

Even though we recommend that you start out meditating in your special place and at your special time, we do so merely to help you develop the habit of meditating. One wonderful thing about meditation is that you can do it anywhere at any time.

Meditation is particularly useful when you feel depressed, upset, or just out of balance. All you need do is find a quiet place and a few free minutes. The place may be your car, the supply room, even a stall in the restroom. Give yourself a quick meditation break, allowing the negative to move out and the peace to move in.

MEDITATIVE VISUALIZATION

Meditative visualization is a tool for bringing you rapidly into a meditative state in your daily life. You can use it in a variety of situations where you want to change your mental and emotional state quickly. For example, you are going in to see an acutely ill patient for whom you have developed a deep affection and you suddenly feel fearful or anxious as you approach the room door. Or, you are about to have an evaluative review with your supervisor, with whom you have less than an ideal relationship.

Just close your eyes for a moment and visualize yourself in deep meditation. Feel the calmness, the peace, the tranquility that you feel in a meditative state. If negative thoughts or feelings intrude, let them float by. Return to your space of peacefulness. Take a deep breath, open your eyes, bring that feeling into what is happening for you in the present.

MONITORING YOUR PROGRESS

It may be helpful for you to start a journal as you begin to incorporate regular meditation into your life. Sometimes you may not notice any perceptible changes as a result of the practice. But if you keep a journal of your thoughts, feelings, relationships, illnesses, dreams, and revelations, you will usually find that there has been positive progress over the months, though you may not have been aware of it.

Another way to become aware of how you are changing is observing how your world is reflecting back to you. People in your life may make comments such as "You look different" or "You seem calmer" or "I don't know what it is, but you seem happier." Also, watch how you react to life's everyday challenges. You may find that as you become more anchored in meditation, you are less annoyed and more patient with the petty details of daily living.

LIVING IN A MEDITATIVE WAY

Mindfulness is a way of moving through your daily life in an eyes-open, meditative state. Doing so enables you to bring the peace and clarity of the meditative state to everything you do and to every interaction in which you engage. You can practice mindfulness as you go about any of your routine activities: eating, walking, washing dishes, and so on. You will find that as you make meditation a part of your daily life, it gradually becomes the way in which you live in the world.

NOTES

1. Wallace, R. K., and Benson, H. "The physiology of meditation." *Scientific American*, vol. 226, no. 2 (Feb. 1972): 84–90.

2. Wallace, R. K., Benson, H., and Wilson, A. F. "A wakeful hypometabolic physiologic state." *American Journal of Physiology*, vol. 221, no. 3 (Sept. 1971): 795–799.

3. Wallace, R. K., Benson, H., et al. "Decreased blood lactate during transcendental meditation." *Proceedings of the Federation of American Society for Experimental Biology*, vol. 30, no. 2 (March–April 1971):376.

4. Orme-Johnson, D. "Autonomic stability and transcendental meditation." *Psychosomatic Medicine*, vol. 35, no. 4 (July–August 1973):341–349.

5. Kiecolt-Glaser, J. K., Glaser, R., et al. "Psychosocial enhancement of immunocompetence in a geriatric population." *Health Psychology* **4** (1985): 24–41.

6. Kiecolt-Glaser, J. K., Glaser, R., et al. "Modulation of cellular immunity in medical students." *Journal of Behavioral Medicine* **9** (1986): 5–21.

7. Borysenko, J. *Fire in the Soul: A New Psychology of Spiritual Optimism*. New York: Warner Books, 1993.

SELECTED BIBLIOGRAPHY

Addington, J., and Addington, C. *The Joy of Meditation*. 6th ed. Marina del Rey, CA: DeVorss, 1990.

Benson, H., and Klipper, M. Z. *The Relaxation Response*. New York: Avon, 1976.

Benson, H., and Proctor, W. *Beyond the Relaxation Response*. New York: Time Books, 1984.

Bloomfield, H., Cain, M. P., Jaffe, D. T., and Kory, R. B. *TM: Discovering Inner Energy and Overcoming Stress*. New York: Dell, 1975.

Chinmoy, Sri. *Meditation: Man-Perfection in God-Satisfaction*. 5th ed. Jamaica, NY: Agni Press, 1984.

Harp, D. *The New Three Minute Meditation*. Oakland, CA: New Harbinger Publications, 1990.

Le Shan, L. *How to Meditate: A Guide to Self Discovery*. 9th ed. Boston: Little, Brown, 1979.

Saraydarian, H. *The Science of Meditation*. 2nd ed. Santa Fe Springs, NM: Stockton Trade Press, 1976.

Breathing: The Essence of Life

THE POWER OF BREATHING

In India, where yoga originated, breathing is associated with *prana* — the life-force of the body, the source of all vitality. From this concept the discipline of *pranayama*, the understanding and control of breathing, was developed. Inspiration is, then, more than just the intake of air. It is the taking in of *prana*. To be inspired is to be filled with life.

The Chinese culture also values the practice of breathing. Proper breathing is associated with the flow of *chi,* or energy, through the meridians. *Tai chi* and other oriental exercise practices and martial arts require slower and deeper breathing.

THE PHYSIOLOGY OF BREATHING

Breathing is predominantly an automatic process. Air is sucked into the lungs by the expansion of the thoracic cavity. Atmospheric pressure fills the lungs through the nose and trachea and lowers the diaphragm. When the chest muscles relax, air is released and the diaphragm returns to its original position.

For the lungs to be fully oxygenated air must move through the bronchi, into the bronchioles, and finally into the hair-like alveoli.

EMOTIONS AND BREATHING

Impulses from the respiratory neurons in the medulla oblongata are responsible for the breathing process. These neurons are affected by many factors, including the emotions.

All thoughts have feeling or emotion attached to them, and these emotions have a direct impact on our breathing. The stress, or "fight or flight," reaction in response to the emotions of fear and anger increases the breathing rate. During times of upset, anxiety, or nervousness, people tend to hold their breath. More subtle emotions also impact the breathing. Involuntary brief changes in the volume and rate of breathing are constantly taking place in response to incoming impressions, internal thoughts, and feelings.

Stressful living leads to bad breathing habits. Due to the effects of stress, most people breathe shallowly from the chest. This does not allow for complete aeration of the lungs nor for efficient oxygenation of the blood. Chronic stress can actually restrict your breathing range —the difference between the circumference of your chest upon inhalation and upon exhalation. Successful competitive athletes have a breathing range of about 15%, while the average healthy adult has a 10% range. Heart patients, on the other hand, have a breathing range of only 2% to 5%. When holding one's breath becomes a chronic response to negative emotions, the body can actually armor itself with connective and muscle tissue that physically constricts the normal expansive capabilities of the chest.

BENEFITS OF BREATHING CORRECTLY

Because of the direct connection between the state of your mind and the state of your breathing, emotions clearly affect your breathing. The linkage, however, works both ways. The state of your breathing can also affect the state of your mind. By practicing correct breathing you can balance your sympathetic and parasympathetic nervous systems and bring yourself into a state of calm and peacefulness.

It is interesting to note that the slower breathing animals are generally less excitable and live longer than do animals with more rapid breathing patterns. Monkeys and hens breathe about 30 times per minute, while tortoises breathe only three times per minute.

It has been shown in humans that slow, deep, abdominal breathing decreases the energy expenditure breathing requires, increases oxygenation of the cells, and improves metabolism and elimination. This way of breathing is the most efficient and also the most beneficial for long-term health.

YOUR BREATHING PATTERN

It is important to determine whether you breathe from your chest or from your diaphragm. To do so, simply place your right hand on your abdominal area and your left hand on your chest. Then, inhale deeply through your nose and pay attention to the movement of your hands.

If your left hand rises more than your right, you are breathing from your chest. If your right hand rises more than your left, you are breathing from your diaphragm.

DIAPHRAGMATIC OR ABDOMINAL BREATHING

Diaphragmatic or abdominal breathing is the most efficient way to breathe. When the diaphragm, the large muscle between your chest and abdomen, is contracted, it moves downward creating a vacuum that draws air into your lungs. This type of breathing takes in about eight times as much air as does chest breathing, allows for adequate oxygenation of the alveoli, and improves venous return of blood to the heart.

Diaphragmatic breathing is the breathing method of choice of singers and practitioners of the martial arts and yoga. One of the easiest stress management tools to learn, it can be engaged in anywhere at any time.

Practicing Diaphragmatic Breathing

Sit comfortably with your back straight, resting your right hand on your abdomen and your left hand on your chest, and close your eyes. Inhale deeply through your nose. Then exhale, contracting your abdominal muscles. Your right hand should rise as you inhale and fall on your exhale if you are breathing from your diaphragm.

Some people find it easier to learn this technique by lying flat on their back. If you have trouble breathing this way, it may be helpful to put a pillow or a book on your abdomen and relax your arms by your sides. Concentrate on your breathing and you will feel the object on your abdomen rise and fall as you learn to breathe from your diaphragm.

Do not be discouraged if this new habit feels uncomfortable at first. Most people have spent their entire lives breathing shallowly from the chest. With practice, diaphragmatic breathing can become your normal way of breathing. You will notice that the more you breathe this way the more balanced and calmer you will feel.

DEEP BREATHING

Deep breathing is an extension of diaphragmatic breathing and is the foundation of all yoga practices. It has three stages: inhalation, retention, and exhalation.

First, inhale through the nose. Then focus your concentration on holding your breath. Finally, release the air consciously, emptying the lungs more fully than you usually do.

To enhance your breathing practice, you may want to concentrate as you inhale on the inspiration of the life force or energy. As you retain your breath, concentrate on being filled with and one with this life force. While you exhale, see yourself releasing all negativity and impurities on both the physical and emotional levels.

A specific ratio has been developed by the yogis for those beginning to practice deep breathing. The ratio is breathing in for one unit of time, holding for four units, and breathing out for two units (1:4:2). Inhaled air contains 21% oxygen, while exhaled air contains only 12%. Retaining the inhaled breath allows for a more efficient diffusion of the oxygen-rich air into the stale air remaining in the lungs. Doubling the exhalation time in relation to the inhalation time expels more air from the lungs, promoting an efficient breathing and oxygenation process.

Practicing Deep Relaxation Breathing

Simply sit in a comfortable position with your back straight and your eyes closed. While you are learning this technique, rest your right hand on your abdomen and your left on your chest, as you did when practicing diaphragmatic breathing.

Exhale completely through your nose, and then inhale deeply. Feel your abdomen filling with air and your right hand rising. Continue to inhale as you fill your chest with air, and note how your left hand rises as your chest expands. Inhale even more, filling your lungs and feeling your collarbone rise.

Hold your breath for as long as is comfortable. Do not be concerned about the 1:4:2 ratio as you do this for the first time.

Exhale in the reverse order from the way you inhaled. Release the air slowly, first from your lungs, then from your chest as you feel the contraction in this area. Lastly, allow the air to be released from your abdomen, contracting your abdominal muscles to expel as much air as possible.

If you become dizzy, light-headed, or short of breath while breathing deeply, just go back to your normal way of breathing. It sometimes takes the body a little time to adjust.

As you become used to this exercise, pay attention to your breathing ratio. Proceed at a pace that is comfortable for you. You may want to start with a breathing ratio of 1:1:1 for inhaling, retention, and exhaling. For example, as you breathe in count to four, hold counting to four, and breathe out counting to four. Next you may want to move to a ratio of 1:2:2 before reaching the recommended breathing ratio of 1:4:2. At the 1:4:2 ratio, breathe in counting to 4, hold for a count of 16, and breathe out to a count of 8.

Just a few minutes of deep breathing will put you in a very relaxed state. Make this exercise part of your daily life, using it whenever you feel stressed, upset, anxious, or nervous.

BREATHING FOR BALANCE

Although most people are not aware of it, the breath naturally alternates between the nostrils. The breath flows primarily through one nostril for about two hours and then shifts to the other nostril for about two hours.

Yogis feel that breathing through the left nostril has a relaxing, cholinergic effect on the body, while breathing through the right nostril produces a stimulating, adrenergic effect. Deliberately practicing alternate nostril breathing is a way of balancing the sympathetic and parasympathetic nervous systems and right- and left-brain activity. It has long been used as a yoga technique for developing concentration.

Practicing Alternate Nostril Breathing

Sit comfortably with your back straight and your eyes closed. Fold the first and second fingers of your right hand into your palm.

Close off your right nostril with your right thumb. Inhale through the left nostril. Close your left nostril with the ring finger of your right hand and retain the breath for whatever time is comfortable for you. Open your right nostril by removing your thumb and exhale.

With the left nostril still closed, inhale through the right nostril. Close off the right nostril with your thumb. Retain the breath. Then open your left nostril by removing your ring finger and exhale.

Repeat this process three to five times. As you become comfortable with it, pay attention to your breathing ratio, working up to 1:4:2. Again, should you feel light-headed or dizzy, return to your normal breathing pattern.

BREATHING TO ENERGIZE

As you have seen, breathing techniques can be used to calm yourself, to reach a state of balance, and to achieve clear thinking. Another breathing technique can be used to energize yourself. By using forceful abdominal exhalations, you can move the breath in such a way that it will increase your energy level. This type of breathing is useful when you are feeling sluggish, tired, bored, or depressed.

Practicing Bellows Breathing

Sit with your back straight and your eyes closed. Inhale and exhale deeply once using diaphragmatic breathing. Inhale again, then forcefully exhale a small quantity of air in short bursts, contracting your abdominal muscles. When the lungs have emptied, inhale and exhale deeply once more. Inhale again and repeat the process for three more rounds.

To complete this practice, inhale and exhale gently three times.

WAYS TO IMPROVE YOUR BREATHING

You can improve the efficiency of your breathing by adding aerobic exercise to your lifestyle. Aerobic conditioning enables your body to extract oxygen optimally from inhaled air while minimizing the energy needed to transfer the oxygen to the bloodstream.

Eating dairy products increases mucus production, which may clog your air passages. Minimizing dairy consumption will maximize your breathing efficiency. Since air pollutants also increase mucus production and damage respiratory tissues, avoid them as much as possible.

BREATHING TO RECENTER

Once you have learned deep relaxation breathing, you can use this technique as a stress-reduction tool during your work day. If you find yourself feeling less than centered and calm, find a quiet place—a restroom, lounge, or locker room—and take a few minutes to breathe deeply and recenter yourself.

SELECTED BIBLIOGRAPHY

Kingland, K. and Kingland, V. *Complete Hatha Yoga: In Philosophy and Practice.* New York: Arco Publishing Company, 1976.

Swami Rama, Ballentine, R. and Hymes, A. *Science of Breath: A Practical Guide.* Homesdale: Himalayan International Institute of Yoga Science and Philosophy, 1979.

Wood, E. *Yoga.* Baltimore: Penguin Books, 1959.

Chapter 9

Aerobic Exercise: The Active Form

AEROBICS

Just as two types of mind exercises—the active visualization and affirmation and the receptive meditation—combine to form a balanced mindcise program, two types of exercises together comprise a balanced physical program. The active form, aerobics, is addressed in this chapter, while the receptive form, yoga, is presented in Chapter 10.

Aerobics literally means "promoting the supply of oxygen." Aerobic exercise involves moving steadily and vigorously over an established time period so that the cardiovascular system works at a rate that demands large amounts of oxygen. Developed by Dr. Kenneth Cooper, director of the Aerobic Center in Dallas, Texas, aerobics is now considered one of the most important methods for attaining fitness.

Though many sports and fitness activities are vigorous, not all are necessarily aerobic. Such stop-and-go sports as doubles tennis, paddle ball, and team volleyball may make the cardiovascular system work hard, but only in short bursts. Your body draws on its nonoxygen, anaerobic system during these short periods of high-intensity exercise. The anaerobic response provides you with quick energy, but also produces large amounts of lactic acid, which may cause muscle soreness and pain. To achieve the training effect of aerobic conditioning, exercise must be steady and sustained.

Fitness

Regular aerobic exercise increases fitness. Fitness is a measure of how efficiently your body can extract oxygen from the blood and transport it to your muscles while you are exercising. Both the number of small blood vessels in your muscles and the number of mitochondria that supply energy inside the muscle cells increase in response to regular aerobic exercise. A fit body is a more efficient body that can do more work with less effort than an unfit one.

BENEFITS OF AEROBIC EXERCISE

Among many benefits of regular aerobic exercise for both the body and the mind are:

1. *Increased longevity.* A number of research studies have demonstrated that men and women who are fit live longer than those who do not exercise (Ornish, Note 1).

2. *Improved heart health.* Aerobics promotes a healthy heart by minimizing coronary disease risk factors. Aerobic exercise reduces blood pressure, decreases blood clot formation, raises the high-density lipoproteins (HDL) or "good" cholesterol, and lowers triglycerides.

3. *Improved bone health.* Bone density is increased with aerobic exercise. This benefit is particularly important for postmenopausal women, who often suffer from osteoporosis and increased risk of bone fracture.

4. *Improved fat burning.* Aerobics helps muscle tissues become more efficient at oxidizing fat. As you age, the percentage of body fat tends to increase, even if your weight remains the same. Also, many people tend to gain weight as they get older. Aerobics can change these tendencies.

5. *Decreased anxiety and depression.* Norepinephrine levels double during aerobics, resulting in the lifting of depression. A number of studies have also noted that people who regularly exercise exhibit less anxiety and have fewer medical complaints than those who do not engage in a routine aerobics program.

6. *Induced relaxation.* One of the best remedies for stress is aerobic exercise. Engaging in physical activity is relaxing and incompatible with maintaining skeletal-muscular tension.

7. *Increased energy level.* Fitter people tend to be more active people. They are generally energetic and feel good about themselves. In contrast, sedentary people often do not like the way they look or feel and may routinely resist activity, fearing that they may tire easily or injure themselves.

HOW MUCH AEROBICS IS ENOUGH?

One interesting finding of the research on fitness and longevity is that you need not spend very much time exercising aerobically to receive the many benefits of doing so. Moderate fitness is associated with increased longevity. Highly fit individuals have slightly increased longevity over their moderately fit peers, but the largest difference in longevity has been seen between those who are sedentary and those who exercise moderately.

Moderate activity of 30 minutes per day or one hour three times per week at conditioning intensity is sufficient to maintain good health and increase longevity.

CONDITIONING INTENSITY

To experience a conditioning or "training" effect from your exercise program, you must engage in your chosen aerobic activity at an intensity level based on your age and your heart rate.

Most exercise experts agree that you need to exercise at between 60% to 80% of your maximum heart rate to achieve a conditioning effect. Several formulas exist for calculating your target heart rate. Figure 9-1 uses the Karvonen Equation, currently recommended by the American College of Sports Medicine.

FIGURE 9-1
Target Heart Rate

Target heart rate = (maximum heart rate − resting heart rate) × (0.60) + resting heart rate
Target heart rate = (maximum heart rate − resting heart rate) × (0.80) + resting heart rate

Maximum heart rate = 220 − your age
Resting heart rate = One-minute pulse at rest (Ten-second pulse × six)

Example: You are 34 years old with a ten-second carotid or radial artery pulse of 14.

Target heart rate = 186 − 84 = 102 × 0.60 = 61 + 84 = 145
Target heart rate = 186 − 84 = 102 × 0.80 = 82 + 84 = 166

You must keep your pulse rate between 145 and 166 beats per minute to achieve a training effect from your exercise.

Monitoring Your Pulse

Take a ten-second pulse and multiply it by six during your exercise routine to ensure that you are exercising within your target range. If your pulse is too slow, exercise a little harder. If it is too high, slow your pace a bit.

Another way of monitoring the intensity of your workout is to see if you can continue talk during the exercise. If you find you do not have enough breath to converse, you are probably overexerting yourself. Ease up and try talking again once you have regained your breath.

TYPES OF AEROBIC EXERCISE

It does not matter which of the many types of aerobic exercise you select. What does matter is that you choose an exercise that you enjoy doing and will thus do consistently.

Consider your social as well as physical needs. If you have a hectic life-style, filled with people day and night, you may want to select an exercise you can do by yourself such as walking, running, or cycling. If, on the other hand, you enjoy the social exchange of exercising with others, you may select an aerobic dance or exercise class, join a health club, or arrange to walk or run with a friend.

Walking

Walking is a low-impact aerobic exercise that can be done anywhere by just about anyone. All you need are comfortable, supportive shoes. A regular walking program builds stamina and endurance and tones the leg muscles. A half hour daily of vigorous walking raises your oxygen consumption level to the point of a cardiovascular training effect and also burns between 180 to 250 calories.

As your body becomes conditioned and your heart more efficient, you will find that you must walk longer or faster to reach your target heart rate. Some alternate jogging with walking will increase the intensity of the exercise to the appropriate level.

Hiking

Hiking is a little more strenuous than walking if you are gaining altitude as you hike. In addition to the conditioning benefits, hiking brings you closer to nature, which in itself is both invigorating and relaxing. Remember that there is less oxygen the higher you go. If you are hiking at 10,000 feet, go slowly the first day or two to allow your body to acclimate.

Running

Running provides the most intense aerobic exercise in the shortest amount of time. Like walking, it can be done just about anywhere. Unless you are already fit, it is best to start a running program slowly and build up gradually.

The best way to start is at a slow jog. As you need more intensity to reach your target heart rate, increase the speed or duration of your run. Running is high-impact exercise and can subject your feet and knees to quite a pounding, so many people prefer to run on a soft, dirt track, in a park, or on the wet-packed sand of a beach. If you experience any pain in your knees or feet, discontinue running until your injuries heal. When you begin again, start out slowly and run on a soft surface.

Bicycling

Bicycling is basically a lower-body activity, producing powerful thighs and long leg muscles. As it is a nonweight-bearing exercise, bicycling is an excellent choice for anyone with chronic joint or foot problems.

Note, however, that bicycling is an aerobic exercise only if it is done correctly. Coasting, though fun, does not produce a training effect. Pumping steadily over a reasonable distance is good aerobic exercise, and cycling over hilly terrain is an excellent way to condition your heart.

If you prefer the environment of a health club, most have computerized, stationary bicycles that you can program to meet your training needs.

Swimming

Swimming is one of the best total body conditioners, putting your body through a nearly stressless but extremely efficient resistance workout. It is a particularly good exercise choice if you are overweight or have joint or injury problems.

Increased endurance, stamina, coordination, and muscle tone are among the many benefits of swimming. To achieve a conditioning effect, you must swim continuous laps for at least 20 minutes.

Aquaexercise classes are also a good aerobic choice, because the buoyancy of the water assists in performing the exercises. Again, this is an excellent choice for individuals who have difficulty in engaging in exercise on a hard surface.

Cross-Country Skiing

Cross-country skiing requires more calories per hour than any other aerobic activity because it demands the use of all the major muscle groups. Combining low-impact activity with high fat burning, cross-country skiing is a true total-body conditioner, building both the upper and lower body and making tremendous demands on the cardiovascular system. When done properly, it is a blend of endurance and grace.

Many health clubs have cross-country skiing machines to allow you to reap the benefits of this sport indoors. Using these machines is also a good way to prepare your body for this winter activity.

Aerobics Classes

Aerobics classes are usually very accessible in most locations. Class options may include high-impact, low-impact, aerobic dance, and stair-step. Low-impact is easier on the joints than are the other options. Aerobic dance or jazz dance classes provide excellent conditioning. Nightclub dancing can also be aerobic if you sustain the activity for an extended period of time.

Conditioning Machines

Most health clubs have aerobic conditioning machines. Choices may include treadmills, stair-steppers, stationary bicycles, and rowing and cross-country skiing machines. Many of these machines are computerized, allowing you to select an intensity of exercise that matches your conditioning requirements. Home versions of most of these machines are also available.

Although the weight-stack machines such as Nautilus and Universal are excellent for building muscle bulk, strength, and endurance, they do not provide you with an aerobic workout.

Videotapes

Many videotapes exist on the market offering instruction in a variety of aerobic activities. Videotapes offer you the advantage of a structured class at any time that is convenient for you and allow you to achieve the full benefits of a health club workout without leaving the comfort of your home.

Daily Activities

If you are a floor nurse, you are probably on your feet and moving a good portion of your workday. There are, however, other ways you can incorporate additional exercise into your daily routine. For example, you can climb the stairs rather than take the elevator. Walking or bicycling to work or the store is better than driving. If time, distance, or weather conditions do not allow you to bike or walk, park your car as far away as possible from the building entrance and walk.

Although being physically active in your daily routine is good, you still need to engage in aerobic activity of sufficient frequency, intensity, and duration to receive conditioning benefits.

AEROBIC PRECAUTIONS

Consult Your Physician

If you are new to exercise, plan on doing more than walking, and are over 35, consult your physician before beginning your exercise routine. This is particularly important if you are overweight, a smoker, or have heart disease, high blood pressure, diabetes, arthritis, or any other medical problem that concerns you.

Always Stretch Before and After

Allow five minutes before and after your aerobic exercise for stretching. Stretching before aerobics increases the flow of blood to the areas stretched. It elongates and reduces the tension in the muscles stretched and increases the range of movement around the joints. Stretching after exercise, while your muscles are still warm, prevents stiffness and increases flexibility.

At a minimum, be sure to stretch the thigh and calf muscles of your legs and do side reaches with your arms. Hold for at least 30 seconds, breathing deeply and slowly as you stretch. This gives the muscle and connective tissue time to stretch productively. Regularly stretching will lengthen the muscles and surrounding tissue, reducing risk of injury.

Avoid Injury

Start your program slowly if you have been sedentary, and then increase your workouts gradually as you get stronger. Jumping in and doing too much too fast may lead to injury. People who engage in high-impact, high-intensity activity of extended duration such as long-distance running may suffer orthopedic injuries. Moderation is the key to success. To avoid injuries and maximize the benefits of aerobic activity, consult the recommendations in Figure 9-2.

CHANGING WEIGHT

Most exercise physiologists and physicians maintain that it may take about three months from the time you initiate a consistent exercise program until you decrease your weight. This is particularly true if you have been sedentary for a long time.

Also, note that muscle weighs more than fat. As you become more muscular, your body will burn fat more efficiently but you may not notice a significant decrease in weight. You will, however, notice that your clothes fit differently as you tighten and tone your muscles.

FIGURE 9-2
Aerobic "Dos"

1. Consult your physician. If you are over 35, overweight, sedentary, or have medical problems, this is an important first step for you.

2. Pick an exercise that you enjoy.

3. Start slowly if you are sedentary. You may need to begin by doing three 10-minute walks or two 15-minute walks to build up to one 30-minute walk.

4. Increase the intensity of your workouts slowly. If after walking for a while you are no longer reaching your target heart rate, do not just start running. Instead, alternate jogging with walking and then build up to jogging the entire distance.

5. Increase the duration of your workouts. As you become more conditioned, extend your workouts by 10- to 15-minute increments.

6. Exercise 30 minutes a day or one hour three times a week to achieve a conditioning effect.

7. Always stretch at least five minutes before and five minutes after your aerobic activity.

8. Some muscle soreness is natural when you begin an exercise program. It takes a little time for your muscles to get used to a new level of exertion. This is a healthy soreness that goes away with repeated activity.

9. Do it!

CREATING AN EXERCISE PLAN

The first step in making exercise a routine part of your life is to create a realistic plan for yourself. Figure 9-3 provides you with a tool for getting started.

List each activity you currently do, the duration of that activity, and any new activity you plan to add for each day of the week. For example, you are now walking 15 minutes on Saturday and Sunday and you add 15 minutes on Monday and Wednesday and 15 minutes to your Sunday walk. If you are currently sedentary, give yourself up to eight weeks to work up to 30 minutes per day or three hours per week.

FIGURE 9-3
Exercise Plan

	Mon.	Tues.	Wed.
Week 1	Now: Add:	Now: Add:	Now: Add:
Week 2	Now: Add:	Now: Add:	Now: Add:
Week 3	Now: Add:	Now: Add:	Now: Add:
Week 4	Now: Add:	Now: Add:	Now: Add:
Week 5	Now: Add:	Now: Add:	Now: Add:
Week 6	Now: Add:	Now: Add:	Now: Add:
Week 7	Now: Add:	Now: Add:	Now: Add:
Week 8	Now: Add:	Now: Add:	Now: Add:

Thurs.	Fri.	Sat.	Sun.
Now: Add:	Now: Add:	Now: Add:	Now: Add:
Now: Add:	Now: Add:	Now: Add:	Now: Add:
Now: Add:	Now: Add:	Now: Add:	Now: Add:
Now: Add:	Now: Add:	Now: Add:	Now: Add:
Now: Add:	Now: Add:	Now: Add:	Now: Add:
Now: Add:	Now: Add:	Now: Add:	Now: Add:
Now: Add:	Now: Add:	Now: Add:	Now: Add:
Now: Add:	Now: Add:	Now: Add:	Now: Add:

NOTE

1. Ornish, D. *Dr. Dean Ornish's Program for Reversing Heart Disease*. New York: Ballantine Books, 1990.

SELECTED BIBLIOGRAPHY

American College of Sports Medicine. *Guidelines for Exercise Testing and Prescription*. Philadelphia: Lea & Febiger, 1986.

Cooper, K. *The Aerobics Program for Total Well-Being*. New York: Bantam Books, 1982.

Meyers, C. *Walking: A Complete Guide to the Complete Exercise*. New York: Random House, 1992.

Yanker, G. *The Complete Book of Exercise Walking*. Chicago: Contemporary Books, 1983.

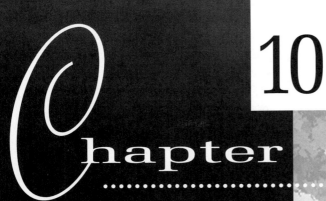

Chapter 10

Yoga Asanas: The Receptive Form

THE RECEPTIVE FORM

In contrast to active exercise such as aerobics, receptive exercise uses breathing and concentration in conjunction with movement. There are various forms of receptive exercise. Tai chi, which originated in China, and yoga, developed in India, are the most well known. Yoga has been selected as the receptive form discussed in this chapter since it is more easily self-taught than tai chi, although both are equally effective.

THE WAYS OF YOGA

Yoga, a Sanskrit word, means "uniting" or "bringing together as one." It is an approach to living a balanced life where body, mind, and spirit are harmonious. Yoga is based on the ancient teachings found in the *Upanishads*, the Hindu spiritual treatises written in 800–400 B.C. and later clarified and classified by Patanjali into eight ways of being, as shown in Figure 10-1.

FIGURE 10-1
The Eight Ways of Yoga

1. *Yama:* Universal moral commandments

2. *Niyama:* Rules for daily conduct

3. *Asanas:* Postures

4. *Pranayama:* Understanding and controlling the breath

5. *Pratyahara:* Understanding and controlling the senses

6. *Dharana:* Concentration of mind on a single point

7. *Dhyana:* Meditation

8. *Samadhi:* Union with the real self

HATHA YOGA

Hatha yoga is a series of gentle stretching exercises using specific *asanas* (postures) and *pranayama* (breathing techniques). Hatha yoga, translated from the Sanskrit, means "sun and moon." Hatha yoga is about attaining and maintaining a state of balance between the sun and moon, the masculine and the feminine, the sympathetic and the parasympathetic, the warm and the cool, the day and the night.

Whereas aerobics focuses on building strength and endurance, hatha yoga focuses on increasing flexibility, grace, and vitality. Yoga teachers in their 60s and 70s consistently look far younger than their years and move with the grace and suppleness of professional dancers. Longtime yoga practitioners are also known for their clarity of mind and levity of attitude.

Physiology of Yoga

Most people have chronically tensed muscles. Studies of athletes have shown that tense muscles impair performance. Today, many professional athletes from a variety of sports are adding flexibility exercises to their routine training because they know that a relaxed and flexible body is a more efficient one.

Hatha yoga is a scientific system of exercises that not only relaxes and tones the muscles, but also has a profound effect on the endocrine and nervous systems. The bending, stretching, and holding properties of the postures, along with the accompanying slow, deep breathing, stimulate the production of endocrine hormones and have a tonic effect on the central nervous system.

The results of regular practice over an extended time period are flexibility, a toned and firm body, vitality, emotional and mental clarity, and peacefulness. Hatha yoga is an important component of Dr. Dean Ornish's successful and highly acclaimed Program for Reversing Heart Disease (Ornish, Note 1).

Yoga and Breathing

Pranayama, or the yoga of breathing, is an integral part of hatha yoga. The type of breathing most commonly used for achieving full benefits from the yoga postures is slow, deep, diaphragmatic breathing. Breathing this way assists you to hold the postures for an extended period and gently increase your stretching, as your body and mind relax into the rhythm of your breathing.

Yoga and Concentration

Hatha yoga is as much a discipline of the mind as it is of the body. Some yoga experts go so far as to say that concentration is 90% of the practice. During the practice of the postures, the mind is focused on breathing and stretching. If your mind wanders or becomes absorbed in the events of your daily life, it needs to be brought back to a state of oneness with the posture.

Balancing postures are a good demonstration of this fact. Many of the balancing postures are not that demanding physically, but they do require intense concentration. You will find that you lose your balance, not because of lack of physical strength, but solely because your mind wanders.

BEGINNING YOUR YOGA PRACTICE

All you need to begin your practice of yoga are comfortable, non-binding clothes and a quiet place. If the place you choose is not carpeted, you will want to use an exercise mat, pad, or beach towel for the sitting and lying postures. It is best to do yoga either first thing in the morning before breakfast or later in the evening, at least two hours after dinner. It is very important to have an empty stomach when you do yoga, as many of the postures place pressure on the intestinal area.

You will find that your body is more flexible later in the day than in the morning. Some people enjoy doing yoga both in the morning and in the evening. Consult Figure 10-2 for additional recommendations.

HOW MUCH YOGA IS ENOUGH?

Most yoga teachers recommend that the beginning student practice 20 to 30 minutes a day. If you have been sedentary for a long time, you may want to start by doing 20 minutes every other day.

There are more than 3,000 yoga postures. In this chapter we describe for you verbally and visually a few of the more common beginning postures. Practicing all of these postures daily is ideal. If you do not have sufficient time to do them all, at least do three sets of the *Sun Salutation*. This one posture, with its 12 parts, is designed as a tonic for all body systems.

FIGURE 10-2
Yoga "Dos"

1. Choose a clean, quiet place for your practice.

2. Practice at the same time(s) every day. It is better to do a little yoga every day than an extended session once a week.

3. Make sure you have not eaten for at least two hours before you begin your practice.

4. Before you begin the postures, take a few slow, deep breaths and clear your mind from the thoughts of the day.

5. Keep your mind focused on your breathing and postures. If your mind should wander during practice, gently push the extraneous thoughts away and focus again on the posture and your breathing.

6. Move slowly and smoothly as you do the postures. Yoga should be done with the grace of ballet, not with the abrupt movements of aerobic dance.

7. Hold each posture for about one minute, but never longer than is comfortable for you. One minute is about ten slow, deep breaths.

8. Always balance a posture that stretches you in one direction with its complementary posture. For example, the forward *Alternate Leg Pull* should be balanced by the *Cobra*, which stretches the back in the opposite direction. The *Shoulder Stand* should always be followed by the *Fish*.

9. As you become more flexible, increase the duration of your stretch in one-minute increments.

10. Never force yourself to stretch further than your body is comfortably willing to go. Yoga works by gradually loosening and relaxing your muscles and increasing the flexibility of your spine and joints. It takes time and repetitive practice to learn how to relax chronically tensed muscles and stiff joints.

11. Do the resting postures whenever you think you may have stretched a little too far or when you feel tired. The two resting postures are the *Child's Pose* and the *Relaxation Pose*.

12. Be patient and gentle with yourself. Yoga changes your body, but gradually, not instantly. You should feel relaxed and energized after doing yoga. This is usually an immediate result for most people. You may find that you can do a posture easily one day, but that you are stiff when you repeat this position for the next few days. Do not be discouraged. Your body is simply adjusting itself to its new way of being. Continued practice will result in increased flexibility and an enhanced sense of well-being.

13. Do it!

YOUR YOGA PLAN

Simply add your yoga sessions to your overall Exercise Plan (see Figure 9-3).

THE YOGA POSTURES

Asana means to hold a position, relaxed and motionless, for a period of time. Become the posture. Feel where your body is loose and where it is tight. Breathe into the tight spots as you continue the stretch. You will find that as you breathe and concentrate your body will relax a little more and you will be able to stretch a little further. Each posture has benefits for specific muscles, organs, and glands.

Neck Rolls

Benefit: Releases tension in the neck and shoulder muscles.

1. Sit on the floor with your back straight and your legs crossed. Close your eyes and inhale.

2. Exhale as you let your chin drop to your chest, or as close to your chest as is comfortable for you. Let your head rest there as you breathe deeply three times.

3. Return your head slowly and gently to its upright position.

4. Inhale as you very slowly let your head drop to the right until your right ear touches your right shoulder. Do not raise your shoulder; simply let the weight of your head gently fall toward your shoulder.

5. Continuing to inhale, move your head from your right shoulder, letting it fall backwards.

6. Beginning to exhale, let your head roll gently toward your left shoulder.

7. Continuing to exhale, let your head roll from your left shoulder to your chest.

8. Gently raise your head to its upright position and take two deep breaths.

9. Repeat the neck roll, moving this time to the left.

10. Do a total of three rolls to the right and three rolls to the left.

11. *Note:* This posture can easily be performed in a chair wherever and whenever you feel tension in your neck or shoulders.

Half-Spinal Twist

Benefits: Improves poor posture; stimulates adrenal glands, kidneys, liver, and spleen; useful to combat constipation and indigestion.

FIGURE 10-3
Half-Spinal Twist

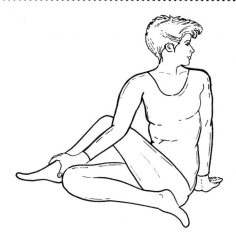

1. Sit on the floor with your back straight and both legs extended.

2. Bend your right knee and position your right foot adjacent to your left buttock.

3. Cross your left leg over your right knee and place your left foot flat on the floor, as shown in Figure 10-3.

4. Raise and straighten your right arm above your head, then place your right palm on your outer left knee allowing it to slide down your calf until you reach your ankle.

5. Extend your left arm behind your buttock, placing your palm on the floor, with the fingers pointed away from your body.

6. Look over your left shoulder, slowly twisting your trunk and head to the left.

7. Take slow, deep breaths as you hold the posture.

8. Slowly untwist and face forward.

9. Repeat on the right side, reversing the placement of arms and legs.

Alternate Leg Stretch

Benefits: Stretches leg and back muscles and spine; stimulates spleen and abdomen; improves digestion.

FIGURE 10-4
Alternate Leg Stretch

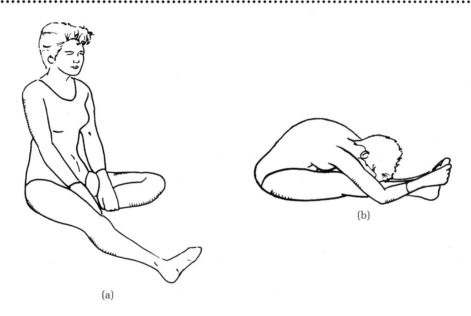

(a)

(b)

1. Sit on the floor with your legs stretched out in front of you and your back straight.

2. Bend your left knee and place the sole of the left foot against the inside of your right thigh, as shown in Figure 10-4(a).

3. Inhaling, lock your thumbs together and raise your hands overhead, stretching your torso as long as you comfortably can.

4. Exhaling, bend forward from the hips, extending your arms toward your right foot while keeping your back straight.

5. Take hold of your right foot, toes, calf, or knee with your hands. It is far more important to keep your back straight than to reach your toes or foot. Extend only as far as is comfortable for you.

6. Hold this position with your head relaxed, breathing slowly and deeply. Figure 10-4(b) shows the maximum stretch.

7. Repeat on the left side.

Cobra (Complement to Alternate Leg Stretch)

Benefits: Stretches spine and spinal nerves; tones back, chest muscles, and genitals; stimulates adrenal glands.

FIGURE 10-5
Cobra

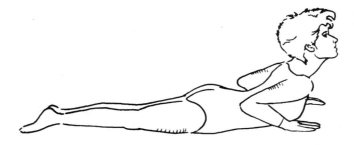

1. Lie on your abdomen with your legs together and your toes pointed straight, as shown in Figure 10-5.

2. Put your palms flat on the floor directly beneath your shoulders, with your elbows raised and close to your body and your fingers pointed forward.

3. Inhale and raise your head, neck and chest slowly off the floor while your pelvis remains on the floor. Lift yourself as high as is comfortable without strain. Hold for 20 seconds.

4. Exhale as you lower your torso slowly, touching your chin to the floor first, then your forehead and finally your shoulders.

5. Turn your head to one side and rest it on your folded arms.

6. Repeat for a total of six times, each time raising your torso a little higher. Upon lowering, rest your head on your folded arms on alternating sides.

Shoulder Stand

Benefits: Stimulates the thyroid and parathyroid glands and gonads; relieves gastrointestinal disorders; beneficial for hernias and varicose veins.

Modified version: If you have back pain, neck or shoulder injuries, or high blood pressure. Lie flat on your back with your hands at your sides. Elevate your feet and legs, keeping your legs straight, and rest your feet on the edge of a chair. Maintain this position, taking deep breaths for two to three minutes.

FIGURE 10-6
Shoulder Stand

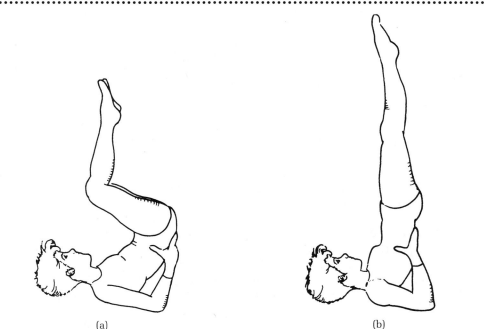

(a)   (b)

1. Lie on your back with your arms at your side and your feet together.

2. Inhale, bend your knees, and raise your torso off the floor by supporting your lower back with your hands and using your upper arms for balance, as shown in Figure 10-6(a).

3. Straighten your legs and get as high up on your shoulders as is comfortable for you, as shown in Figure 10-6(b).

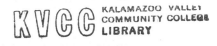

4. Tuck your chin into your chest and hold this position for at least one minute, breathing deeply and slowly. Gradually, work up to holding this position three to five minutes for optimal stimulation of the glands.

5. Exhale as you lower your body, vertebra by vertebra, back to the floor.

Fish (Complement to Shoulder Stand)

Benefits: Stimulates thyroid, parathyroid, pituitary, and pineal glands; stretches neck muscles and cervical and sacral spine.

FIGURE 10-7
FISH

1. Lie on your back with your legs together and your arms at your side.

2. Arch your back, supporting yourself with your elbows, and place the top of your head on the floor, as shown in Figure 10-7.

3. Balance your weight between your head, your elbows, and your buttocks. Breathe deeply as you hold the position.

4. Shift your weight to your elbows, slowly unarch your back, and lift your head off the floor.

5. Lie on your back with your arms at your sides and breathe deeply twice.

Sun Salutation

Benefits: This 12-position posture (see Figure 10-8) is traditionally practiced at dawn as a moving meditation to greet the sun and the beginning of the new day. It improves circulation and stimulates the nervous system while toning the entire body.

This posture can be done at a quicker pace to warm and stimulate the body, or at a slower pace for a cooling and calming effect. Unlike the previously described postures, in this one you move from one position to another without holding any of the positions for an extended period. If you do not have time to do a full yoga routine, do only the *Sun Salutation*, as it is a total body balancer.

FIGURE 10-8
SUN SALUTATION

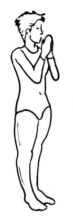

Figure 10-8. Position 1

1. Stand up straight and relaxed, with your feet together and your arms at your sides. Inhale, bringing your hands together at your chest. Exhale.

Figure 10-8. Position 2

2. Lock your thumbs together, stretch your arms in front of you, and inhale. Bend backwards, slightly arching your back, and raise your arms above your head.

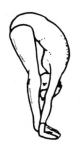

Figure 10-8. Position 3

3. Exhale as you slowly fold your body forward with your legs straight, and place your hands flat on the floor on the outer side of each foot. (Bend your knees slightly if necessary.)

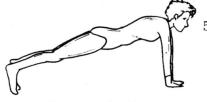

Figure 10-8. Position 4

4. Keeping your hands in the same position, inhale and bend your left knee. Extend your right leg back, with your knee and toes on the floor. Look up and arch your back.

Figure 10-8. Position 5

5. Bring your left leg back parallel to your right leg. Keep your arms straight, pushing into the floor with your hands. Raise yourself off the floor, keeping your entire body straight, and hold your breath.

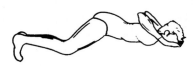

Figure 10-8. Position 6

6. Begin to inhale and lower your knees to the ground, bending your elbows and touching your chest and forehead to the floor. Your pelvis will be slightly lifted, your palms flat on the floor beneath your shoulders, and your elbows close into your body.

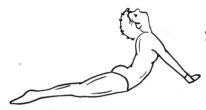

Figure 10-8. Position 7

7. Continuing to inhale, keep your hands in the same position, straighten your arms, lower your pelvis to the floor and stretch your chest, neck, and head upwards, arching your back.

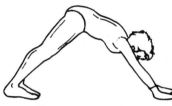

Figure 10-8. Position 8

8. Exhale as you straighten your legs, placing your feet flat on the floor. Maintain your arm position and lift your buttocks to form a triangle.

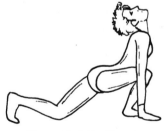

Figure 10-8. Position 9

9. Inhale, keep your hands in the same position, and bend your right knee. Extend your left leg back, with your knee and toes on the floor. Look up and arch your back.

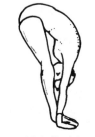

Figure 10-8. Position 10

10. Bring your left leg forward to meet your right and straighten your knees. Exhale as you slowly fold your body forward with your legs straight, and place your hands flat on the floor on the outer side of each foot.

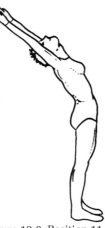

Figure 10-8. Position 11

11. Slowly stand up, lock your thumbs together, and stretch your arms in front of you, inhaling. Bend backwards, slightly arching your back, and raise your arms above your head.

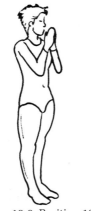

Figure 10-8. Position 12

12. Stand up straight and relaxed, with your feet together and your hands together at your chest. Inhale, letting your arms relax at your sides. Exhale and note how your body feels.

Repeat the twelve-step exercise, this time extending your left leg back in Position 4 and bending your left knee in Position 9. Repeat the complete exercise, alternating right and left, three times.

Child's Pose (Resting Posture)

Benefits: Rest and relaxation.

This pose can be done whenever you feel you need a rest from the other *asanas.* It is also a good relaxation tool you can use whenever you feel tense or stressed.

FIGURE 10-9
Child's Pose

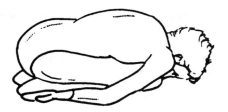

1. Kneel with your legs together and sit on your legs as you inhale.

2. Exhale as you slowly lower your head to the floor in front of your knees. Rest your arms with the palms up adjacent to your legs, as shown in Figure 10-9.

3. Breathe deeply and stay in this position as long as you desire.

Relaxation Pose (Resting Posture)

Benefits: Deep rest and relaxation. Like the *Child's Pose*, this posture is to be used in between more demanding positions or any time you are feeling tense. Yoga sessions usually end with this posture.

FIGURE 10-10
Relaxation Pose

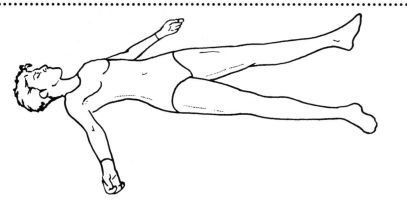

1. Lie flat on your back with your arms comfortably by your sides, hands facing palms up, and feet about 18 inches apart.

2. Tense each part of your body starting at your toes and working up

to your head. Inhale as you contract each body part and exhale as you release it. Visualize all the tension leaving your body.

3. Breathe slowly and deeply, visualizing new energy coming in and bathing your entire body.

ADDITIONAL YOGA RESOURCES

Most large cities have yoga classes, either at a specialized yoga center or at a health club. A class can be a useful adjunct to your daily practice, as the instructor can watch you and gently correct your posture if necessary.

If you do decide to take a class, make sure that the instructor is grounded in a spiritual perspective. Particularly at the health clubs, you may find yoga instructors who are really aerobics instructors and are unaware of the appropriate breathing and pacing of the postures.

Yoga videotapes are also available for home use, and some large cities broadcast yoga programs on the local public television station.

NOTE

1. Ornish, D. *Dr. Dean Ornish's Program for Reversing Heart Disease.* New York: Ballantine Books, 1990.

SELECTED BIBLIOGRAPHY

Feuerstein, G., Bodian, S., and Staff of *Yoga Journal. Living Yoga: A Comprehensive Guide for Daily Life.* New York: Jeremey P. Tarcher/Perigee, 1993.

Hittleman, R. *Richard Hittleman's Yoga: 28 Day Exercise Plan,* 23rd ed. New York: Bantam Books, 1988.

Kingsland, K., and Kingsland, V. *Complete Hatha Yoga: In Philosophy and Practice.* New York: Arco Publishing Co., Inc., 1976.

Robin, M., Nagaranthna, and Nagendra, *Yoga for Common Ailments.* New York: Simon & Schuster, Inc., 1990.

Wood, E. *Yoga.* Baltimore: Penguin Books, 1959.

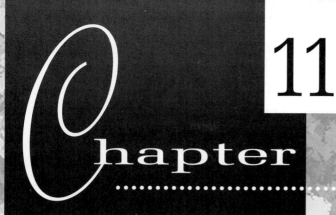

Chapter 11

Massage:
For Healing
and
Relaxation

HISTORY OF MASSAGE

Massage is an ancient healing technique. Roman and Greek physicians used massage as one of the principal means for alleviating pain and healing the body. Hippocrates listed rubbing as a requisite skill of the physicians he trained. Swedish massage, established in the early 1800s, combined knowledge of physiology and gymnastics culled from the Chinese, Egyptian, Greek, and Roman techniques. The oriental systems of massage, acupressure in China and shiatsu in Japan, originated more than 5,000 years ago.

Among today's many different massage techniques, some are more physically oriented, such as Swedish, deep tissue, and rolfing, and others are more energetically oriented, such as shiatsu, acupressure, and reflexology.

BENEFITS OF MASSAGE

Touch is the first sense to develop. Babies initially learn about their world through tactile experience. Experiments with primate and human infants have shown detrimental effects on normal development when nurturing touch is withheld. As humans, we have an innate need to touch and be touched. Although the particular manner of fulfilling this need varies depending on the technique utilized, the touch of massage provides benefits for mind, body, and spirit.

On a physical level, massage can relax and tone the muscles, release lactic acid buildup from exercise, assist the flow of blood and lymph, stretch the joints, and alleviate pain and congestion. Massage can also facilitate the release of body toxins and stimulate the immune system, increasing resistance to disease.

On a mental and emotional level, massage can relieve anxiety and stress, release restrictive emotional patterns that constrict the body, and provide an overall sense of deep relaxation and well-being.

Spiritually, massage affords a sense of harmony and balance. When the spiritual aspects of massage are emphasized, you may experience a state of deep meditation and a shift in perceptions that remains after completion of the massage. You may, as a result, gain a fresh perspective on your true nature and your place in the universe.

KNOWING YOUR BODY

Before beginning a session, massage therapists usually ask if clients would like to concentrate on any problem areas. Often the client cannot specify these areas. When they do, the designated areas are frequently far less needy than are other areas of which clients are totally unaware.

Most people are not aware of where they carry tension. One way to access this information is by body scanning.

Body Scanning

Body scanning is a tool for learning where you are carrying tension in your body. If you have recently started an exercise program and have sore muscles, do not take them into consideration during this process. Instead look for chronic holding patterns that may create an acute reaction for you under stress. Follow the process step by step, making mental notes of tense or sore spots. Record your findings on the Body Scan Checklist in Figure 11-1 after completing the process.

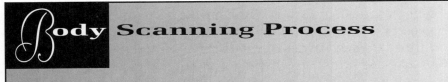

ody Scanning Process

Set-up: Find a quiet environment free of sounds or light. Lie on your back on the floor with knees bent and your feet flat. Review the following instructions first and then close your eyes. You will palpate different areas of your body to identify your personal tension spots. Be sure to apply sufficient pressure with your fingers as you explore your body.

1. **Head:** Move both hands to the top of your head, pressing the crown. Separate the two hands, pressing the right side with your right hand and the left side with your left hand. Next, gently turn your head to the right and feel the back left portion of your skull with your left hand. Finally, turn your head to the left and press the right back portion of your skull with your right hand. When finished, return your head to center.

2. **Neck:** With your head resting on the floor, palpate each side of your neck with the corresponding hand. Move both hands to the

back of the neck, proceeding from the lower portion of your neck to the area where the neck joins the head.

3. **Shoulders:** Feel each shoulder, both front and back, with the opposite hand. Press fairly deeply with a circular motion into these areas.

4. **Face:** Start from your forehead working down. Palpate the bones under your eyebrows and then proceed to the area beside both eyes and the bones beneath them. Then move to the area of the cheekbones adjacent to your nose. Finally, explore the jaw areas on each side of your face.

5. **Chest:** Palpate your entire chest, paying particular attention to the area between your breasts.

6. **Abdomen:** Palpate your entire abdominal area, starting below your breast bone and moving down to the groin.

7. **Arms and hands:** Using the hand from the opposite side of the body, proceed to feel for any tender spots in your arms, starting from your upper arm and working down to your wrists. Take time to palpate the elbows. Probe the palms of your hands; and flex each finger away from the palm.

8. **Legs:** Bend your knees so that your feet are resting flat on the floor. Move down each leg with both hands, making sure to palpate the knees. Then proceed down the calves to the ankles.

9. **Lower back:** Turn over and lie on your stomach with your entire body flat on the floor. Starting at your waist, move your hands down either side of your spinal cord until you reach the tip of the tailbone. Starting at the tailbone, feel the areas between your spine and your hips, moving up to the waistline.

10. **Buttocks and hips:** Explore your buttocks and hips for sore spots. Use firm pressure in these areas.

FIGURE 11-1
Body Scan Checklist

Check any areas where you felt soreness or tension during the scanning process:

___ *Head*

___ Right side ___ Left side ___ Back

___ *Neck*

___ Right side ___ Left side ___ Back ___ Connection with head

___ *Shoulders*

___ Right front ___ Left front ___ Right back ___ Left back

___ *Face*

___ Forehead ___ Eyebrow bones ___ Side of eyes

___ Cheekbones ___ Jaws

___ *Chest*

___ Right side ___ Left side ___ Between breasts

___ *Abdomen*

___ Upper right ___ Lower right ___ Upper left ___ Lower left

___ *Arms and hands*

___ Right arm ___ Left arm ___ Right hand ___ Left hand

___ *Legs*

___ Right upper ___ Left upper ___ Right calf ___ Left calf

___ *Lower back*

___ Right side ___ Left side

___ *Buttocks and hips*

___ Right buttock ___ Left buttock ___ Right hip ___ Left hip

___ *Other* (elaborate)

Symptom History

Another way to know your body and its reaction to stress is to assess symptoms you are currently experiencing or have experienced in the past when you have been stressed. Take a few minutes to complete your stress symptom history in Figure 11-2.

FIGURE 11-2
Stress Symptom History

SYMPTOM	CURRENT	PAST
Headaches	_____	_____
Eye pressure	_____	_____
Jaw pain/Tightness	_____	_____
Neck pain/Stiffness	_____	_____
Shoulder pain/Stiffness	_____	_____
Abdominal tension		
Pain	_____	_____
Diarrhea	_____	_____
Constipation	_____	_____
Gas/Bloating	_____	_____
Butterflies/Queasy	_____	_____
Leg cramps	_____	_____
Insomnia	_____	_____
Excessive sleeping	_____	_____
Others:	_____	_____
_____	_____	_____
_____	_____	_____
_____	_____	_____

SELF-MASSAGE

Although receiving a massage from someone else is wonderful, it is not always convenient or feasible to do so. Fortunately, massage techniques exist that you can use yourself to release specific pains and tensions or to help yourself relax. Two of these techniques, acupressure and foot reflexology will be presented in Chapters 12 and 13, respectively.

SELECTED BIBLIOGRAPHY

Downing, G. *The Massage Book*, 34th ed. New York: Random House, 1992.

Lawrence, D. B. *Massage Techniques*. New York: Putnam Publishing, 1986.

Lidell, L. *The Book of Massage: The Complete Step-by-Step Guide to Eastern and Western Techniques*. New York: Simon & Schuster, 1984.

Malstrom, S. D. *Own Your Own Body*. New Canaan, CT: Keats Publishing, 1977.

Tappan, F. *Healing Massage Techniques: Holistic, Classic and Emerging Methods*. Norwalk, CT: Appleton & Lange, 1988.

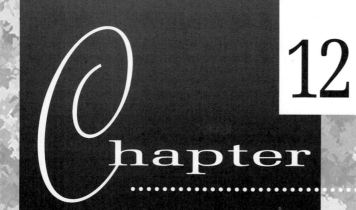

Chapter 12

Self-Massage: Acupressure

ACUPRESSURE

Acupressure, originated in China, is the ancient healing art of applying finger pressure to specific locations on the body. Whereas acupuncture uses needles to stimulate energetic points, acupressure activates the same points by pressure.

Chinese medicine considers local symptoms to be an expression of imbalance in the bodymind as a whole. Treatment is aimed not only at relieving the symptoms, but at reestablishing a state of health and harmony in the body, mind, and spirit.

How Acupressure Works

The Chinese have identified a series of channels running longitudinally on the body called *meridians*. These pathways are conduits for the body's circulating energy, or *chi*. Each pathway is associated with particular organs and psycho-physical functions. For example, the liver meridian is associated not only with the liver, but with the nails, muscles, tendons, reproductive system, eyes, the emotion of anger, and the ability to plan.

The meridians and their abbreviations are: Lung (**Lu**), Large Intestine (**LI**), Stomach (**St**), Spleen (**Sp**), Heart (**H**), Small Intestine (**SI**), Bladder (**B**), Kidney (**K**), Pericardium (**P**), Triple Warmer (**TW**), Gallbladder (**GB**), Liver (**Lv**), Governing Vessel (**GV**), and Conception Vessel (**CV**). The various acupressure points are located on their respective meridians. These areas are particularly sensitive to bioelectrical impulses in the body.

More than three hundred acupressure points have been charted and related to specific symptoms. Some points relieve more than one symptom, particularly when they are stimulated in conjunction with other associated points. Each point is named for its position on a specific meridian. For example, **GB 20** refers to a point on the gallbladder meridian, while **LI 14** specifies a point on the large intestine meridian. When acupressure points are stimulated, they allow the flow of the body's energy to treat the condition under consideration.

The points are not always located adjacent to the area of the body to which they are responsive. For example, a point in the back of the knee relieves lower back pain and sciatica. And points in the web between the thumb and first finger on the hands alleviate headaches.

Stimulating acupressure points triggers the release of endorphins, the natural pain-reducing neurochemicals. The flow of energy, blood, and oxygen is increased and muscle tension decreases. With energy flowing freely, the body can come to a healthy balance.

ACUPRESSURE SELF-MASSAGE

Acupressure self-massage involves the stimulation of a pattern of acupressure points on your own body.

Self-Acupressure Mechanics

The middle finger and the thumb work best for self-acupressure because they are the strongest fingers. Some treatment points, however, require using two or three fingers or, in some cases, your fist in a particular area. For those patterns that specify using your fingers, you may use your knuckles or fist if your fingers hurt or feel too weak. Pencil erasers, golf balls, or other hard, small objects may also be used.

Pressure should be applied gently and slowly at first, and then gradually and firmly increased. The pressing finger or thumb should be held at a 90 degree angle to the surface of the skin, and the pressure should be firm enough so that you feel it.

If you press a point that is extremely tender, ease up on the pressure until you can handle the sensitivity of that point. A sensitive point indicates a congestion of energy that needs treatment. If you breathe deeply and slowly as you hold the point, you will find that the tenderness decreases rapidly.

Hold the point until the pain diminishes or you feel a pulsation in the point, generally about two to three minutes. The pulsation is an indication that the blockage has been released and the energy is again flowing. When you have finished holding the point, release your finger slowly, encouraging the continuation of the newly established energy pattern.

ACUPRESSURE TREATMENT PATTERNS

Acupressure self-massage is effective for a variety of conditions. Treatment patterns for some common stress-related complaints are provided in the sections that follow.

Shoulder Tension

Shoulder tension, a very common symptom, may result from repetition of occupational activities that strain the shoulders. Emotionally, shoulder tension is associated with feeling burdened by responsibilities you are carrying—or "shouldering."

If you have this symptom, you will experience immediate relief from working the points described below. However, because shoulder tension is usually a chronic condition accumulated over a long period of time, it may take several acupressure sessions to release your shoulders totally. Sit comfortably in a chair while implementing the pattern described here and illustrated in Figure 12-1.

FIGURE 12-1
Shoulder Tension

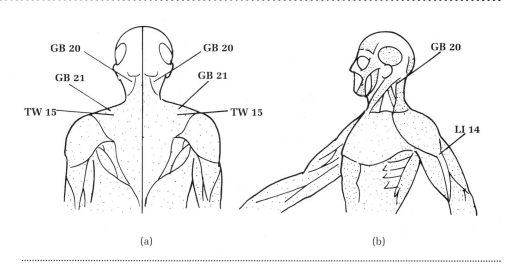

(a)   (b)

Point Locations

Point Location: TW 15
One-half inch below the top of the shoulders, midway between the base of the neck and the outer extreme of the shoulders.

Point Location: GB 21 *(Do not press if pregnant.)*
The highest point of this shoulder muscle, one to two inches from either side of the base of the neck.

Point Location: LI 14
On the upper arm, one-third of the way between the shoulder and the elbow, on the muscle adjacent to the bone on the outer side of the arm.

Point Location: GB 20
In the hollow, approximately two to three inches wide, between the two large vertical neck muscles below the base of the skull.

Treatment Sequence

1. Curve the fingers of both hands, placing them over the tops of each shoulder on **TW 15**. Apply pressure, using your first three fingers, allowing the weight of your relaxed arms to increase the pressure applied to your shoulders. Breathe deeply as you hold these points.

2. Put the first three fingers of your right hand on the top of your left shoulder on **GB 21**. At the same time, place the first three fingers of your left hand on the outside of your upper right arm on **LI 14**. Press both points at the same time, taking deep breaths. Gradually increase the pressure on your shoulder muscle as it relaxes and softens. Then press both **GB 21** and **LI 14** on the other side the same way, breathing slowly and deeply.

3. Insert your thumbs in the indentations at the base of your skull at **GB 20** and close your eyes. Tilt your head back slowly as you press up and under the skull, gradually increasing the pressure. Breathe deeply as you hold these points.

Neck Tension and Pain

Located between the seat of the mind and the body, the neck tends to become tense when there is an imbalance between the two. A common experience when the body is tired is that the mind will not still itself. Neck tension and pain are often also related to repressing the expression of your true feelings. The following pattern, designed to alleviate these symptoms, should be done seated, referring to Figure 12-2.

FIGURE 12-2
Neck Tension

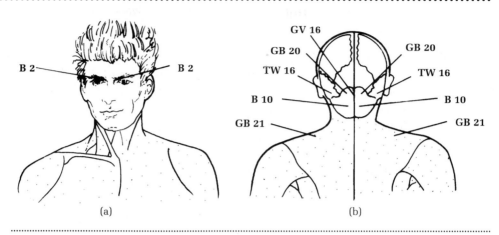

(a)   (b)

Point Locations

Point Location: GB 21 *(Do not press if pregnant.)*
On the highest point of this shoulder muscle, one to two inches from either side of the base of the neck.

Point Location: B 10
On the ropy muscles one-half inch away from the spine and about one-half inch below the base of the skull.

Point Location: TW 16
One to two inches behind each earlobe in the indentation at the base of the skull.

Point Location: GB 20
In the hollow, approximately two to three inches wide, between the two large vertical neck muscles below the base of the skull.

Point Location: GV 16
In the large hollow under the base of the skull in the center of the back of the head.

Point Location: B 2
Where the bridge of the nose meets the inner ridge of the eyebrows at the indentation of each inner eye socket.

Treatment Sequence

1. Hook the first three fingers of each hand on **GB 21** at the top of each shoulder. Relax the arms, allowing the weight of the arms to increase the pressure of your hands hooked on **GB 21**.

2. Curving your first three fingers once again, place them on **B 10**, applying firm pressure to the points on the ropy muscles of your neck. Inhale, raising your head slowly, and then exhale, lowering your head toward your chest. Repeat this movement slowly three times. Then with your head slightly lowered, continue holding the points until the pain decreases or pulsation begins.

3. Place your thumbs in the indentations at **GB 20** under the base of your skull, closing your eyes and breathing deeply. On releasing **GB 20**, slide your hands toward your earlobes, slipping your thumbs into the **TW 16** indentations. As these points are often sensitive, take care to increase the pressure you apply gradually. Then hold steady pressure on these points while breathing slowly and deeply.

4. Place your left thumb in **GV 16** in the large hollow under the base of the skull. At the same time, using the thumb and index finger of your right hand, press on **B 2** of each eye socket. Press upward, breathing deeply.

Headaches

Headaches can be caused by many factors. Most result from muscle tension in the head, neck, and shoulders which constricts the blood vessels supplying the head. This muscle tension is usually associated with anxiety, worry, or stress. Misaligned cervical vertebrae can cause certain headaches, as can constipation, often related to frontal headaches. A buildup of fluid pressure in the sinus cavities can also cause headaches. The following acupressure pattern, illustrated in Figure 12-3, can help alleviate these types of headaches. You should be either seated or lying down as you engage in this pattern.

FIGURE 12-3
Headaches

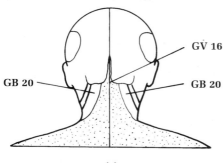

(a)

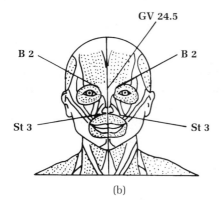

(b)

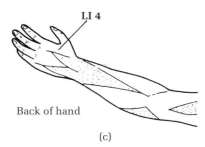

Back of hand

(c)

Point Locations

Point Location: GB 20
In the hollow, approximately two to three inches wide, between the two large vertical neck muscles below the base of the skull.

Point Location: GV 16
In the large hollow under the base of the skull in the center of the back of the head.

Point Location: B 2
Where the bridge of the nose meets the inner ridge of the eyebrows, at the indentation of each inner eye socket.

Point Location: GV 24.5
Between the eyebrows where the bridge of the nose meets the forehead.

Point Location: St 3
At the bottom of each cheekbone adjacent to the nose and in line with the pupil of each eye.

Point Location: LI 4 *(Do not press if you are pregnant.)*
At the highest spot on the muscle in the webbing between the thumb and index finger.

Treatment Sequence

1. Place your thumbs in the **GB 20** indentations beneath the base of the skull. While pressing these points, slowly tilt your head backwards with your eyes closed and take long, deep breaths.

2. Place your left thumb in **GV 16** in the large hollow under the base of the skull. At the same time, using the thumb and index finger of your right hand, press upward on B 2 of each eye socket, breathing deeply.

3. Put your two palms together, pressing **GV 24.5** between your eyebrows with the index fingers of both hands. Let your head tilt forward and breathe deeply.

4. With your head remaining in a tilted position, use the index and third finger of both hands to press **St 3** beneath the cheekbones in direct line with the pupil of each eye as you continue your deep breathing.

5. Placing your right hand over the top of your left, apply pressure with your right thumb to the highest spot, **LI 4**, in the webbing between your left thumb and index finger. If you can not find the spot right away, probe that area until you find a point that is tender. Pressing this point, take long, slow breaths. Repeat this procedure, applying pressure to your right hand.

Backaches

Backaches are another very common ailment. The majority of back problems are related to stress, weak abdominal muscles, poor posture, or accidents. If there is no inflammation in the back, the effects of acupressure can be increased when used in conjunction with heat in the form of a hot bath, hot water bottle, or heating pad. The acupressure pattern for lower back problems, illustrated in Figure 12-4, is initiated in a seated position and completed lying down.

FIGURE 12-4
Backaches

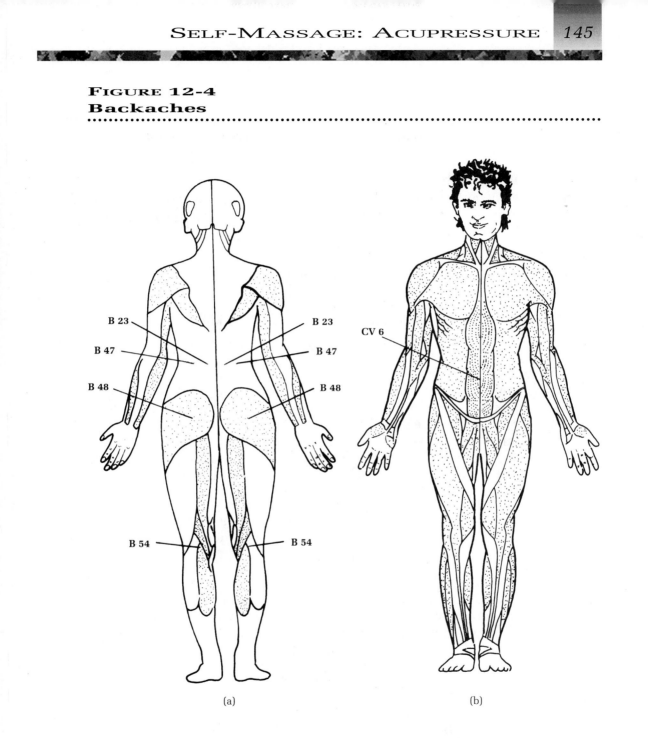

B 23

B 23

B 47

B 47

B 48

B 48

CV 6

B 54

B 54

(a)

(b)

Point Locations

Point Locations: B 23 and B 47

The area two to four fingers away from the spine laterally, at waist level (between the second and third lumbar vertebrae).

Point Location: B 48

Midway between the top of the hipbone and the base of the buttock and one to two finger widths laterally from the large bony area at the base of the spine (the sacrum).

Point Location: CV 6

Two finger widths directly below the belly button.

Point Location: B 54

In the center of the crease at the back of the knee.

Treatment Sequence

1. Sitting on a stool or on a chair facing its back, place the knuckles of both hands on your lower back at the level of your waist with your palms facing out. Rub your back briskly with your knuckles to create warmth. Breathe deeply as you do this. Then place your hands on your waist and use your thumbs to press first the outer point, **B 47**, and then the inner point, **B 23**. Apply as much pressure as you can without causing discomfort and keep breathing deeply.

2. Lying on your back with your legs extended flat on the floor, place the index finger of each hand two finger widths directly under your belly button on **CV 6** and press deeply into the abdomen while breathing.

3. Still lying down, bend your knees so that your feet are flat on the floor. Place your hands with palms downward and fingers pointing toward your feet beneath the center of your buttocks. With your eyes closed and breathing deeply, rock your knees slowly from side to side, stimulating **B 48**.

4. Still on your back, bend your knees toward your chest and press your index fingers into **B 54**, at the center of the crease behind your knees. Using your arm muscles to help, rock your body forward and backward, breathing slowly and deeply as you do so.

5. Lying on your back with your knees bent and your feet flat on the floor, make fists and position them at waist level under **B 23** and **B 47** with the knuckles pressing against your back and the palms

facing down. Let the weight of your body rest on your knuckles. Close your eyes and breathe deeply.

Constipation

Constipation is a fairly common reaction to stress and may also result from lack of exercise, insufficient fiber in the diet, or inadequate intake of water. Often accompanied by gas, bloating, and abdominal pain, constipation can cause headaches if not relieved. Perform this pattern, illustrated in Figure 12-5, while lying on the floor.

FIGURE 12-5
CONSTIPATION

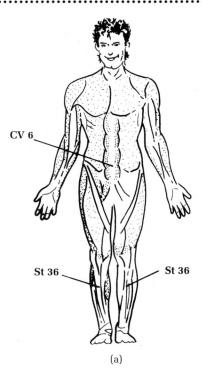

(a)

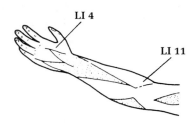

(b)

Point Locations

Point Location: CV 6
Two finger widths directly below the belly button.

Point Location: St 36
One finger width from the shinbone toward the outer side of the leg and four finger widths below the kneecap.

Point Location: LI 4
At the highest spot on the muscle in the webbing between the thumb and index finger.

Point Location: LI 11
On the outside edge of the elbow crease.

Treatment Sequence

1. Lying on your back with your legs extended flat on the floor, place the index finger of each hand two finger widths directly under your belly button on **CV 6** and press deeply into the abdomen while breathing slowly.

2. Still lying on your back, place a rolled towel or pillow under your right knee. Press your right heel into **St 36**, briskly rubbing the point and breathing deeply. Switch legs and repeat the procedure using the left heel.

3. Placing your right hand over the top of your left, apply pressure with your right thumb to the highest spot, **LI 4**, in the webbing between your left thumb and index finger. If you cannot find the spot right away, feel around in that area until you find a point that is tender. Hold this point and take long, slow breaths. Repeat the procedure to your right hand.

4. Still lying down, bend the elbow of your right arm and relax your right hand, palm down, onto your chest. Press firmly with your left index finger into the indentation on the outer edge of the crease of your right elbow, **LI 11**, and breathe deeply. Repeat this procedure on your left arm.

5. Lie on your back with your knees bent and your feet flat on the floor. Imagine a circle beginning three finger widths above your belly button and extending to right above your pubic bone. Using the index fingers of both hands, move clockwise pressing into your abdominal area every couple of inches, slowly and firmly, while breathing deeply. Repeat this procedure slowly three times, continuing to breathe deeply as you do so.

Anxiety and Nervousness

Anxiety and nervousness can be circumstantially related to temporary stressors in your environment, or they may be your way of being in the world. As deep breathing is a disperser of anxiety, it is most important to concentrate on your breathing as you engage in this pattern. Referring to Figure 12-6, perform this pattern while seated, preferably in a chair with arms.

FIGURE 12-6
ANXIETY AND NERVOUSNESS

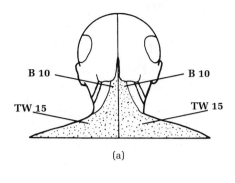

(a)

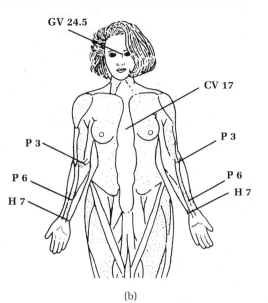

(b)

Point Locations

Point Location: TW 15
One-half inch below the top of the shoulders, midway between the base of the neck and the outer side of the shoulder.

Point Location: B 10
One-half inch outward from the spine and one finger width below the base of the skull on the ropy muscles.

Point Location: P 3
The indentation on the inside of the bent arm at the innermost edge of the elbow crease.

Point Location: P 6
Two and one-half finger widths from the wrist crease, in the middle of the inner side of the forearm.

Point Location: H 7
In the crease of the wrist on the little finger side.

Point Location: GV 24.5
Between the eyebrows where the bridge of the nose meets the forehead.

Point Location: CV 17
On the center of the breastbone, three thumb widths up from the bone's base.

Treatment Sequence

1. Curve the fingers of both hands and place them over the top of each shoulder on **TW 15**. Apply pressure using your first three fingers, allowing the weight of your relaxed arms to increase that pressure. Breathe deeply as you hold these points.

2. Hook the index fingers of both hands onto **B 10** on the ropy neck muscles. Press firmly, breathing deeply and slowly.

3. Relax your arm, bending it at the elbow and resting it on the chair armrest. Press **P 3** on the inside of the elbow crease with your thumb, breathing slowly. Repeat on the other arm.

4. Continuing to rest your arm on the armrest, press **P 6** and **H 7** at the same time, using your index and third fingers. As you do so, take long, slow breaths. Repeat on the other arm.

5. Put your two palms together and press **GV 24.5** between your eyebrows with the index fingers of both hands. Let your head tilt forward and breathe deeply.

6. With your palms still together, move your hands down to your heart area and press firmly against **CV 17** on your breastbone. Really concentrate on your breathing here, letting each breath be a little slower, longer, and deeper than the previous one.

SELECTED BIBLIOGRAPHY

Gach, M. R. *Acupressure's Potent Points: A Guide to Self-Care for Common Ailments.* New York: Bantam, 1990.

Jarmey, C., and Tindall, J. *Acupressure for Common Ailments.* New York: Simon & Schuster, 1991.

Kaptchuk, T .J. *The Web That Has No Weaver.* New York: Congdon & Weed, 1983.

Kenyon, J. *Acupressure Techniques: A Self-Help Guide.* Rochester, NY: Healing Arts Press, 1988.

Teeguarden, I. M. *The Joy of Feeling: Bodymind Acupressure.* Tokyo: Japan Publications, 1987.

Chapter 13

Self-Massage: Foot Reflexology

REFLEXOLOGY

Reflexology, like acupressure, is an ancient healing art. Depicted in detail in Egyptian wall paintings dating from approximately 2300 B.C., it is believed to have evolved a few thousand years earlier. Reflexology's modern origins can be traced to an American physician, Dr. William H. Fitzgerald, in the early 1900s. Fitzgerald's major contribution to reflexology was his definition of distinct vertical zones of energy in the body. By applying pressure to certain parts of the fingers, Fitzgerald discovered he could relieve pain in other body parts located within the same vertical energy zone.

Eunice Ingham is credited with the establishment of reflexology in its present form. In the 1930s she discovered that feet were more responsive to treatment than fingers and developed reflexology treatment patterns for the feet. Her work is carried on today by the International Institute of Reflexology, founded in 1973.

Reflexology is based on the principle that the hands and feet are mirrors of the body and that they have reflex points that correspond specifically to each of the body's organs, structures, and glands.

The body, according to reflexology theory, is divided into ten zones running longitudinally from the head to the feet, with five zones on each side, one corresponding to each of the five toes. When the energy flow through these zones is impeded, disease can result. Stimulating blocked or congested reflexes can release the stagnation, returning the body to a state of optimal health.

The main benefit of reflexology is the release of stress and tension in the body. When the body returns to a state of harmony, circulation and nervous system function are improved.

FOOT REFLEXOLOGY

Since the feet have been found to be more responsive to reflexology than the hands, they will be our focus for describing the practice of self-reflexology. Figures 13-1(a), (b), and (d) chart the major reflexes. Note in part (c) of this figure how the foot reflexes depicted represent an accurate portrayal of the body.

FIGURE 13-1
Foot Reflexology Charts

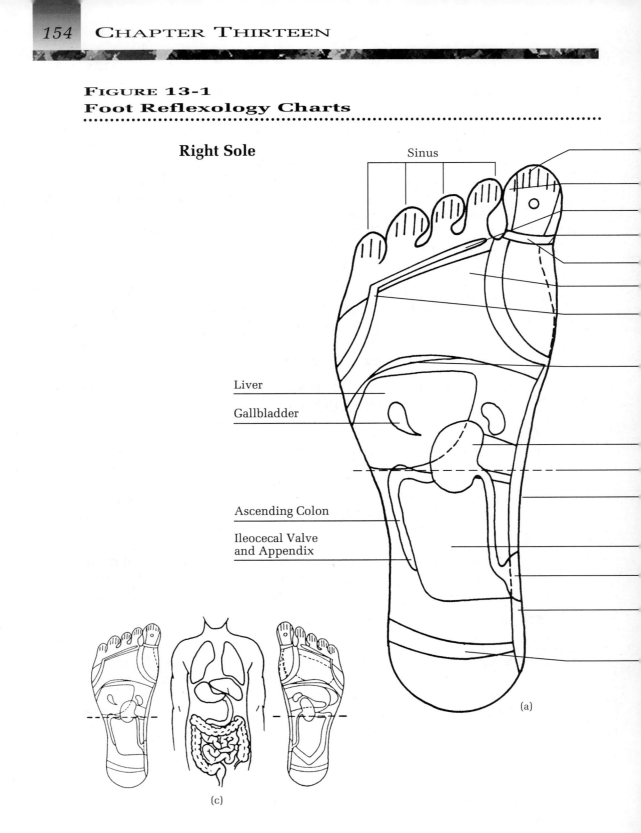

Right Sole

Sinus

Liver

Gallbladder

Ascending Colon

Ileocecal Valve
and Appendix

(a)

(c)

Left Sole

Brain

Side of Neck

Eyes/Ears

7th Cervical

Throat/Neck/Thyroid

Lungs

Shoulder

Heart

Diaphragm/Solar Plexus

Stomach

Kidneys

Waist Line

Spine

Descending Colon

Small Intestine

Bladder

Sacrum/Coccyx

Sigmoid Colon

Sciatic

Sinus

(b)

Right Outside

Hip/Back/Sciatic

Ovary/Testicle

Hip/Knee/Leg

Arm/Shoulder

Lung

Sinus

(d)

FOOT REFLEXOLOGY SELF-MASSAGE

As a nurse you are probably on your feet for most of your working day. Giving yourself a foot reflexology treatment is a wonderful way to relax at the end of your shift. Because the treatment can be done anywhere, you may also want to give yourself one during a break or your lunch hour.

A few preliminary cautions are in order here. Do not use foot reflexology if you have varicose veins or if you are pregnant. Stimulation of the reflexes is very powerful and may have adverse effects in these situations.

Giving Yourself a Treatment

The only equipment you need to do a self-reflexology session is a comfortable chair with a back. You will be pressing spots on the soles and tops of your feet with your thumbs and first fingers, using firm steady pressure.

There are two approaches to reflexology treatment. If you have a particular problem, you can find the reflex area corresponding to your problem on the foot chart and work on that area. For example, if you are having digestive problems, press the areas on the foot that correspond to the stomach, ascending and descending colon, the small intestine, and the ileocecal valve. You may also want to work with the **Gallbladder** and **Liver Reflexes**.

The other approach is to give yourself an overall treatment, identifying those parts of your body that are out of balance as you are working. Finding a sore spot indicates that this area and the associated organ, structure, or gland need work. Continue pressing the spot, breathing deeply as you work on it. Release the reflex when the pain begins to diminish. Totally relaxing a reflex may take a few sessions.

GENERAL SELF-REFLEXOLOGY SESSION

The general pattern is to work on the reflexes systematically from the top of the foot down to the bottom. Refer to the foot charts to identify the reflexes on which you are working.

Treatment Pattern

1. Place your right foot on your left knee, turning the bottom of your foot toward you. Cradle the top of your right foot in the palm of your left hand.

2. Place your right hand on top of your toes and gently rock your foot back and forth several times.

3. Still holding your toes and cradling your foot, rotate your foot slowly clockwise. Repeat this motion several times. Then reverse direction and rotate your foot counterclockwise.

4. Cradling your foot in your left hand, begin to work the **Brain and Sinuses Reflexes**. Move your right hand to the top of the left edge of your large toe. Press this toe with your right thumb on the bottom side and your right index finger on the top side. Keep pressing, moving from the top of the toe to the junction with the sole. Repeat this procedure starting at the middle top of the big toe and moving downward. Then repeat it again working on the right edge of the toe.

5. Repeat the procedure described in Step 4 for each of your toes, starting on the left edge, proceeding to the middle, and concluding with the right edge.

6. With the foot still cradled, walk along the **Eye and Ear Reflexes** with your right thumb, starting on the inside of the foot and working outward. Then reverse direction, walking your thumb from the outside to the inside of the reflex area.

7. Using your right thumb, work around the **Neck and Throat Reflex** on the base of the big toe, working from left to right and then reversing the direction.

8. To work the **Lung Reflex**, hold the right toes with your left hand. Use the outside corner of your right thumb to work up between each of the bones from the bottom of the **Lung Reflex** to the base of each toe, starting with the baby toe and ending with the big toe. Then work downward from the base of each toe to the bottom of the reflex.

9. Continue to hold the toes with your left hand. Press the **Liver Reflex** with your right thumb, moving from right to left, dropping down slightly, then moving from left to right. Continue this pattern until you complete this large reflex area.

10. Next, still holding the toes, use your right thumb to work the **Ascending Colon**, **Ileocecal Valve**, and **Appendix Reflexes** moving from the lower area upward.

11. Cradling your foot in your left palm, work the **Spinal Reflex** on the inside edge of the foot. Starting at the bottom with the coccyx/sacrum area, press with your right thumb. Work up through the lumbar and thoracic area and end with the cervical area at the top of the foot.

12. Hold your foot upright with your left hand and use your right index finger to work the **Hip/Knee/Leg Reflex**, starting from the area near the outside of the heel and moving toward the toes. See Figure 13-1(d).

13. Switch feet, putting your left foot on your right knee, and repeat the pattern described in the preceding steps. Note that the left foot differs from the right in the abdominal area, with the **Stomach**, **Descending Colon**, and **Small Intestine Reflexes** replacing those for the **Liver**, **Ascending Colon**, **Ileocecal Valve**, and **Appendix Reflexes**.

SELECTED BIBLIOGRAPHY

Byers, D. C. *Better Health with Foot Reflexology*. St. Petersburg, FL: Ingham Publishing, Inc., 1983.

Dougans, I., and Ellis, S. *The Art of Reflexology*. Rockport, MA: Element, 1992.

Marquardt, H. *Reflex Zone Therapy of the Feet: A Textbook for Therapists*. Rochester, NY: Healing Arts Press, 1984.

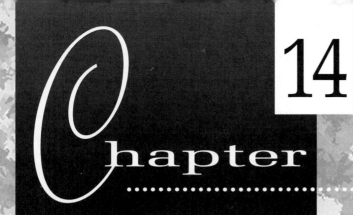

Chapter 14

Nutrition: The Basics

CHANGING AWARENESS

In recent years public awareness about nutrition has increased. A major turning point in this level of consciousness came about with the 1988 release of *The Surgeon General's Report on Nutrition and Health*, in which Dr. C. Everett Koop, recognized dietary intake as a causal factor in heart disease, cancer, stroke, diabetes, atherosclerosis, hypertension, obesity, dental disease, osteoporosis, and gastrointestinal disease. The report identified saturated fat and cholesterol as the main dietary contributors to these problems.

Following the publication of this report, the recommendations of voluntary health organizations, and further medical research documenting the importance of nutrition in both health maintenance and disease prevention, the availability of healthier food products in supermarkets and restaurants has increased exponentially.

Although you may have an interest in eating for health rather than simply for pleasure, you may not have easily accessible, accurate information or the self-awareness and motivation required to change long-standing behavior patterns.

This chapter and Chapters 15 and 16 are designed to provide you with the most current information available and to increase self-awareness of your eating habits and relationship to food. This chapter begins with an overview of basic nutritional concepts. Although this information may be familiar to you, a review of these principles serves as a foundation for concepts discussed in the next two chapters and for building a healthy eating style.

HOW YOUR BODY PROCESSES FOOD

The foods you eat are chemically complex and must be broken down by your body into simpler forms. Once in usable forms, they can be transported to the cells, where they provide energy and the correct building materials for maintaining a healthy body. This process has three steps: digestion, absorption, and metabolism.

Digestion

Digestion is a series of chemical and physical reactions that prepare the food you have eaten for absorption from the intestinal tract into the bloodstream. These reactions are mediated by enzymes in the salivary glands, stomach, pancreas, and wall of the small intestine.

The salivary glands moisten the food you chew with saliva. Saliva contains ptyalin, the enzyme that breaks down carbohydrates. Peristalsis, a wavelike motion of the digestive tract, moves the food into the middle portion of the stomach. Here the food is mixed with hydrochloric acid, enzymes, and water which together break down proteins and other complex substances.

The food, now in the form of liquid chyme, continues by peristalsis to move from the stomach into the small intestine. Carbohydrates move most quickly followed by protein; fat takes the longest time to move through the system.

Once the chyme is in the small intestine, additional digestive processes take place. The pancreas secretes a variety of enzymes, collectively known as pancreatic juices, and the hormone insulin. If fats are present, the liver secretes bile to assist in their digestion and to prepare them for the additional action of the pancreatic enzymes.

Any remaining undigested products enter the large intestine or colon. From here they are eliminated by excretion, with only water being absorbed back into the colon.

Absorption

After food has been completely digested, it is in usable form for absorption. Carbohydrates have been transformed to glucose, protein to amino acids and fat to fatty acids and glycerol.

These nutrients are absorbed primarily in the small intestine through small fingerlike projections called villi. The villi contain both capillaries and lymph channels. Fat is moved directly through the lymph system to the cells, while the other nutrients are funneled from the capillaries into the portal vein leading to the liver.

The liver does a sorting process, utilizing a variety of enzymes to convert the nutrients into new forms for specific purposes. Some of these nutrients move into the bloodstream and then into the cells. The liver uses other nutrients for its own functions and stores still others for later use by the body.

Metabolism

Metabolism is the process of converting the digestive nutrients either into energy or into components needed to build or maintain living tissue. This process is mediated by a complex and extensive enzyme system, which facilitates the thousands of different chemical reactions involved and controls the rate at which these reactions occur.

Metabolism occurs simultaneously as anabolism and catabolism. Anabolism encompasses all the chemical reactions involved in using nutrients for the construction of body tissues and the production of vital chemicals such as enzymes, hormones, and blood. Catabolism includes all the reactions involved in the breakdown of nutrients for the release of energy; this process primarily involves glucose, although energy can also be obtained from fatty and amino acids when necessary.

A New Eating Standard

The average American diet is about 25% to 35% carbohydrates, 25% proteins, and 40% to 50% fats, most of which are saturated. Government agencies and organizations such as the American Heart Association, the National Cholesterol Education Program, the National Research Council, and the new FDA Rules and Regulations for food labeling recommend that fat consumption comprise 30% or less of total calories.

Although the recommended limit of 30% or less is a step in the right direction, epidemiological studies have shown that populations who live long, productive lives free of degenerative disease and obesity obtain about 75% to 80% of their calories from complex carbohydrates, 10% to 15% from proteins, and only 10% from fats. This standard was first heralded by nutritional pioneer Nathan Pritikin. Today, other leaders, such as Dr. Dean Ornish, use these nutritional guidelines in programs for preventing and reversing degenerative diseases and premature aging.

Achieving this new standard may take you a little time, particularly if you subsist on hamburgers and fries. Just start from where you are and incorporate these healthier eating habits into your lifestyle little by little. Moving from a 50% fat and 35% protein diet to a 30% fat and 25% protein diet, for example, is a big step in the right direction.

You will find that as your body adapts to this new way of eating, you will feel more energetic, have better bowel function, and move toward an optimal weight. Cravings for your old favorite foods will diminish over time, and temptations to revert to your old ways will become fewer.

Complex Carbohydrates

The mainstay of this new way of eating is complex carbohydrates, commonly known as starches. Complex carbohydrates are found in such foods as whole grains, vegetables, legumes (beans), and fruits.

High in fiber and valuable nutrients such as vitamins, minerals, proteins, and enzymes, complex carbohydrates are an efficient source of fuel for the body, utilized by the brain, nervous system, and muscles. Complex carbohydrates also assist in the digestion of fats and proteins. High in fiber, a predominantly complex carbohydrate diet facilitates healthy bowel function, increasing stool bulk and toxin release.

Complex carbohydrates are a wonderful aid to proper weight maintenance. They are very filling due to their high fiber content, and since they require much more energy to digest and metabolize than does fat, only a small portion of the complex carbohydrates consumed are converted into body fats.

Another important source of carbohydrates for healthy eating are foods containing cellulose, which provides bulk and assists in elimination.

Protein

Protein is the second most plentiful substance in the body. It is the major source of building material for the internal organs, muscles, blood, skin, hair, and nails, and is important for maintaining good health and vitality.

Recent nitrogen balance studies, however, show that the human body requires far less protein than was previously believed. Studies by the World Health Organization report that the body requires merely 4½% of total calories be protein, while the National Research Council recommends 8%.

Excessive protein intake results in toxic byproducts that can cause great damage to the body. Bone demineralization and osteoporosis are directly linked to excess protein consumption. Other conditions correlated with high-protein diets are arthritis, kidney disease, and liver dysfunction. Many forms of cancer are linked to both high protein and high fat intake.

Protein is built from amino acids. In addition to the 13 amino acids synthesized by the body, nine other essential amino acids must be obtained from food. Your primary protein source should be from the vegetable rather than the animal kingdom since vegetables are far lower in fat than are animal foods.

Plant Protein

Unlike animal protein, plant protein, with few exceptions, does not contain all essential amino acids in any one source. Therefore, a variety of sources of plant proteins must be combined to ensure the availability of all necessary amino acids. The easiest way to obtain the full complement of amino acids is to combine whole grains and beans, including soybean derivatives such as tofu, tempeh, miso, and soymilk, or members of the bean family listed in Figure 14-1. These need not be eaten together in a single meal, but merely consumed sometime during each 24-hour period. The staple foods of many indigenous cultures are beans and grains.

FIGURE 14-1
Common Legumes

Adzuki	Mung
Black	Navy
Black-eyed peas	Peas
Garbanzo	Pinto
Kidney	Red
Lentils	Soybeans

Combining whole grains and small amounts of skim milk or nonfat yogurt is another way to obtain a balanced complement of plant protein. However, if you have lactose intolerance symptoms such as gas or bloating, or any kind of breathing difficulty such as asthma or allergies, avoid dairy products, as they create mucus.

Whole grains are grains that have not been stripped by processing of their highly nutritive germ and bran. Figure 14-2 lists the most common. Whole grains are particularly rich in Vitamins E and the B-complex and in beneficial omega-3 (EPAs) fatty acids. Amaranth from Mexico and quinoa from Peru are fairly new in the U.S. marketplace. These grains were reputed to have been the staple food source of the Mayans and the Incas, respectively, during the time those cultures flourished and were reputed to have provided exceptional energy to the natives who consumed them. Whole grains must usually be purchased in health food stores, although many supermarkets now stock brown rice and buckwheat.

FIGURE 14-2
Whole Grains

Amaranth	Quinoa
Barley	Whole Oats
Brown Rice	Whole Rye
Buckwheat (toasted)	Whole Wheat
Millet	Wheat Berries

Nuts are a good source of plant protein; however, they are also very high in both monounsaturated and polyunsaturated fat and calories, and they are not easily digested. Nuts and nut butters should not be included in the diet if you are carrying excess weight or tend toward constipation. Otherwise, they should be included only in moderation.

Many good vegetarian cookbooks are available to assist you in creating appetizing, healthful meals. In a 1988 position paper, the American Dietetic Association acknowledged that an adequately planned vegetarian diet is healthful and nutritionally sound. They also noted in this same paper the relationship between a vegetarian diet and reduced risk of obesity, coronary artery disease, hypertension, diabetes mellitus, cancers of the lung, breast, and colon, osteoporosis, kidney stones, gallstones, and diverticular disease.

Animal Protein

If you do want to include animal protein in your diet, limit your intake to no more than three ounces per day, two to three times a week. Ocean fish other than shellfish, such as salmon, is the best protein source, as it is rich in omega-3 oils, which help protect the heart. Skinless white chicken and turkey meat are also acceptable choices. Egg whites are also a low-fat source of protein.

Fat

Fats, or lipids, are the most concentrated form of dietary energy, with one gram of fat providing nine calories as contrasted to four calories from a gram of carbohydrates or protein. Fats perform many functions in the body. They are carriers for the fat-soluble vitamins, A, D, E, and

K; assist in calcium metabolism; protect and hold the organs in place; and insulate the body from environmental temperature changes.

The average person needs about 14 grams of essential fatty acids daily for proper functioning of the body. However, the typical daily intake is more than 100 grams. This excessive dietary fat leads to immune system dysfunction and degenerative diseases. Excess fat consumption has been linked to obesity, heart disease, many types of cancers, diabetes, arthritis, multiple sclerosis, and cataracts.

All fat is made up of three components: saturated fat, polyunsaturated fat, and monounsaturated fat. Saturated fat is fat that is solid at room temperature. Animal foods are high in saturated fat. Most vegetable foods are low in saturated fat with the exception of coconuts, olives, cocoa and cocoa products such as chocolate, and palm and cottonseed oils. Saturated fats are converted by the liver into cholesterol, and excess cholesterol increases your risk of heart disease. Each year nearly 600,000 people in the U. S. die from heart disease, the leading cause of all deaths.

Oils

Fats that are liquid at room temperature are called oils. They contain varying proportions of saturated, polyunsaturated, and monounsaturated fats. Canola, safflower, sunflower, and olive oils contain less saturated fat than other vegetable oils. Canola has the lowest amount of saturated fat and the highest amount of omega-3 fatty acids, and is low in polyunsaturates. It is the least detrimental of all commercially available oils.

It is important to be aware that all vegetable oils are fats containing some portion of saturated fat. And saturated fat increases cholesterol levels. The reason that cholesterol levels fall when you switch from butter to olive oil is not that olive oil lowers your cholesterol. Rather, it is due to the fact that olive oil simply has less saturated fat than does butter.

Margarines, shortening, and other hydrogenated oils are simply vegetable oils that have been chemically altered to contain more saturated fat. Hydrogenation extends product shelf-life, but none of these products are health promoting.

Consuming vegetable oils high in polyunsaturates is also detrimental, as these oils increase triglyceride levels, compromise the immune system, and increase the risk of cancer and stroke.

Beware of salad bars. They can be deceiving. The raw vegetables are good choices, but be careful about pasta and other predressed salads, and choose your dressings wisely. Remember that one tablespoon of oil contains about 14 grams of fat—equivalent to the total amount your body requires for the entire day.

Cholesterol

Cholesterol, a fat-like material, is a necessary component of cell membranes and a precursor of many steroid hormones and bile salts. Your liver manufactures 75% of the cholesterol needed by your body for its synthesis activities. Under stress, your body produces additional cholesterol.

The other source of cholesterol is the food you eat. Animal foods contain cholesterol, and the saturated fats in the foods you eat are converted to cholesterol by your liver.

Cholesterol has two main components: high-density lipoprotein (HDL) and low-density lipoprotein (LDL). HDL, commonly known as "good cholesterol," transports excess LDL out of the body. LDL, commonly known as "bad cholesterol," is the one that collects as arterial plaques and increases risk of heart disease. Optimal total cholesterol levels, based on the most recent research and epidemiological evidence, are now defined as 150 or 100 plus your age. The optimal ratio of total cholesterol to HDL is 3.0 or less.

Essential Fatty Acids

The essential fatty acids, collectively known as Vitamin F, are linoleic, linolenic, and arachidonic. These fatty acids are important in organ respiration, formation of membranes, lubrication of body cells, glandular activity, blood coagulation, and breakdown of arterial plaque.

When 2% of the total calories in the diet are linoleic, the body is then able to synthesize the other two fatty acids. The best sources of essential fatty acids are whole grains and flax, sesame, sunflower, and pumpkin seeds. Flax seed is the best source of linoleic acid.

Water

Water, the primary component of the body and a necessary ingredient for all body functions, is the most commonly ignored nutrient. Adequate water intake is essential for removing toxins from the kidney and bowels and for maintaining proper muscle tone.

Inadequate water intake leads to water retention and is counterproductive to weight loss. When the kidneys are unable to function efficiently due to insufficient water intake, the liver takes over some of the kidneys' detoxification functions. The liver then metabolizes less fat, and the excess fat remains in the body. Drinking eight glasses (two quarts) of water each day optimizes detoxification, fat metabolism, and excretion of excess sodium. Since overweight people have increased metabolic demands, they should add one extra glass of water daily for each 25 pounds of excess weight.

It is best not to consume water with your meal, as this dilutes nutrients and decreases saliva production and digestive efficiency. Allow one hour before and after a meal as a margin for drinking water or any other beverage. Drinking a couple of glasses of water an hour before eating is a good weight reduction strategy, as doing so creates a feeling of fullness.

YOUR RELATIONSHIP WITH FOOD

Each individual has a unique relationship with food. That relationship can be a complex one, interweaving childhood upbringing, cultural background, emotional coping patterns, self-esteem issues, and lifestyle habits.

Many people have less than a healthy relationship with food. In the U.S. people tend to overeat. The high incidences of heart disease and some forms of cancer are directly related to dietary excesses. At the other end of the spectrum are the diseases of undercomsumption related to perfectionist upbringing and low self-esteem—anorexia and bulimia.

Take a few minutes to complete the checklist in Figure 14-3. The items you check identify behavior patterns that indicate that your personal relationship with food and eating may be less than ideal. Identifying unhealthy patterns is the first step. Changing them is the next. Consult Chapter 6 for mindcise tools to assist you in changing any behaviors that are not health promoting.

FIGURE 14-3
You and Food

1. ___ I always eat three meals a day, even if I am not hungry.

2. ___ I eat more when I am alone than when I am with other people.

3. ___ I like to snack on sweet or salty foods.

4. ___ I eat when I am upset.

5. ___ I keep food with me, in my desk or in my car.

6. ___ I snack in the evening while I watch T.V.

7. ___ I eat in locations other than the dining room or kitchen when I am home.

8. ___ I eat while I am engaging in other activities.

9. ___ I have been known to go on food binges.

10. ___ I eat at social occasions when everyone else is eating, even if I am not hungry.

11. ___ I frequently eat fatty foods such as ice cream, butter, cheese, cream sauces, and so on.

12. ___ I snack while I am cooking.

13. ___ I always clean my plate.

14. ___ I eat when I am stressed.

15. ___ I eat when I feel depressed.

16. ___ When I avoid dealing with my real feelings, I have a tendency to eat.

17. ___ I always feel that I am fat no matter how thin I really am.

18. ___ I am never satisfied with the size of my body.

19. ___ I binge and then vomit to prevent gaining weight.

20. ___ I eat very little because I always feel fat.

HEALTHY EATING

A healthy relationship with food is one in which food is seen as a source of nourishment for sustaining and maintaining the body. Food is eaten only when you are hungry, and the foods you select to eat are those that are beneficial for your health and long-term well-being. The experience of eating is a pleasurable activity in which the textures, aromas, and taste of foods are enjoyed, but neither particular foods nor the act of eating are addictive or constitute substitutes for emotional responses.

Appropriate Quantities

More and more evidence suggests that less is best. Dr. Roy Walford of UCLA, Dr. Edward Masoro of the University of Texas, and others have performed research studies on animals showing that those who consume fewer calories can live 50% longer than those that are not on restricted diets. The animals also showed reduced signs of aging and decreased incidences of cancer, cataracts, and diabetes. It appears that by reducing the demands of processing food, the body is able to metabolize what it does take in more efficiently and with less stress on the organs.

The yogis advise their students to eat no more at one sitting than you can hold when you cup your hands together. This ancient wisdom seems to correlate quite well with the more recent animal studies.

Chewing and Chewing and Chewing

Hippocrates said: "Drink your food and chew your liquid." This statement makes sense when we look again at the physiology of digestion. The digestion of carbohydrates starts in the mouth with the secretion in the saliva of ptyalin. The more food is chewed, the smaller the food particles become and the more ptyalin is secreted.

With adequate chewing, the work of the stomach, intestines, and pancreas is made easier, and elimination becomes more efficient. Chew your food 20 to 30 times until it becomes mush. If you have a tendency to overeat, you will find that when you chew your food adequately you will eat less.

Chewing is particularly important when eating foods containing cellulose. Cellulose, found in such salad foods as lettuce, celery, and cucumbers, is a nonsoluble fiber which remains undigested by any of the enzymes synthesized by the human body. If chewed properly, cellulose acts as a kind of intestinal broom. However, if it is not chewed

FIGURE 14-4
NUTRITIONAL DIARY

	MON.	TUES.	WED.
Breakfast			
Food			
Drink			
After breakfast			
Food			
Drink			
Lunch			
Food			
Drink			
After lunch			
Food			
Drink			
Dinner			
Food			
Drink			
After dinner			
Food			
Drink			

THURS.	FRI.	SAT.	SUN.

sufficiently, it can create blockage in the intestines, resulting in gas, bloating, and gastric discomfort.

Eating as a Relaxing Ritual

Eating should be done in a relaxed way. Food should be eaten slowly and chewed well. Meals should be an enjoyable ritual, whether you eat with others or alone. You may want to create a comforting meal-time environment by lighting candles or playing your favorite music.

When you eat, eat. Do not engage in other activities at the same time. And do not eat when you are stressed or upset. When your body is in a stressed mode, very little energy remains to be directed toward the digestive organs.

Grazing Versus Three Squares

Grazing, or eating small amounts throughout the day, has become quite a popular eating style for many people. Adopted in response to the demands of a busy lifestyle, grazing often becomes a style of choice.

Grazing is actually a healthy way to eat, as consuming small amounts of food throughout the day maintains the blood sugar at a steady level. It is thus a recommended eating style for those with hypoglycemia. Grazing also decreases the tendency to overeat, which you are most likely to do when you are very hungry and have had to wait for some time for the next scheduled meal. If you are a grazer, remember to eat in a relaxed, slow manner.

If you eat three meals a day, it is advisable to make your evening meal the lightest of the day. Evening is the time when most people tend to be less active and therefore require less food to maintain the body functions. Eating a lighter meal in the evening also provides you with more energy, since less energy is being expended on digestion.

EATING DIARY

Most of us are unaware of all that we consume during a day, and what our eating pattern looks like over a week's time frame will usually come as quite a surprise. The first step in determining how your eating pattern compares with an optimal pattern is to do a self-assessment for one week. Record everything you eat and drink, including water, during the course of one week in the Nutritional Diary provided in Figure 14-4. We advise making copies of the blank diary, as you may want to monitor yourself from time to time in the future.

SELECTED BIBLIOGRAPHY

American Dietetic Association. "Position of the American Dietetic Association: vegetarian diets—technical support paper." *ADA Reports.* (1988);88:352–55.

Dunne, L. J. *Nutrition Almanac*, 3rd ed. New York: McGraw-Hill, 1990.

Guyton, A. C. *Physiology of the Human Body*, 6th ed. Philadelphia: Saunders, 1984.

Koop, C. E., *The Surgeon General's Report on Nutrition and Health: Summary and Recommendations* (DHHS publication #88-50211). Washington D.C.: U.S. Public Health Service, Office of the Surgeon General, Department of Health and Human Services, 1988.

Lappe, F. M. *Diet for a Small Planet*, 10th anniversary ed. New York: Ballantine Books, 1982.

Ornish, D. *Dr. Dean Ornish's Program for Reversing Heart Disease.* New York: Ballantine Books, 1990.

Ornish, D. *Eat More, Weigh Less.* New York: HarperCollins, 1993.

Robertson, L., Flinders, C., and Ruppenthal, B. *The New Laurel's Kitchen.* Berkeley: Ten Speed Press, 1986.

Robbins, J. *Diet for a New America.* Walpole, MA: Stillpoint Publishing, 1987.

Scott, M. and Scott, J. *Bean, Pea and Lentil Cookbook.* Yonkers: Consumers Union of the United States, 1991.

Shulman, M. *Fast Vegetarian Feasts: The Revised Edition with Fish.* New York: Doubleday, 1986.

Tracy, L. *The Gradual Vegetarian.* New York: Dell Publishing, 1985.

Walford, R. L. *The Retardation of Aging and Disease by Dietary Restriction.* Springfield, IL: Charles C Thomas, 1988.

Foods That Heal, Foods That Harm

In general, a diet high in complex carbohydrates and low in protein and fat promotes health and prevents disease. There are, however, specific foods that are particularly helpful for immunity and the prevention of degenerative diseases, and others that are detrimental.

FOODS THAT HEAL

Immune Enhancers

Weaknesses in the immune system create a variety of problems, from increased susceptibility during the winter cold and flu season, to allergies, to more serious diseases such as AIDS and cancer.

Foods rich in Vitamins C, E, A, beta-carotene, B-6, B-12, and folic acid support optimal immune function (see Figure 15-1). Adequate intake of zinc, selenium, iron, calcium, magnesium, and manganese is also important.

Free Radical Scavengers

Oxygen free radicals, a byproduct of respiration, are highly energized molecules containing an unpaired electron that are capable of causing molecular damage to DNA, proteins, carbohydrates, and lipids. Free radical damage is associated with cancer, heart disease, brain damage, arthritis, cataracts, emphysema, and aging.

Under normal conditions a balance exists between free radicals and the antioxidants that neutralize them. However, exposure to environmental stresses can tip that balance in a negative direction. Air pollutants, radiation, ultraviolet light, pesticides, industrial solvents, and even some medicines and anesthetics produce free radicals. To combat such stresses, increased intake of foods rich in antioxidants is required.

Antioxidant nutrients include Vitamins A, C, E, and beta-carotene. The minerals zinc, copper, manganese, and selenium are necessary precursors for antioxidant enzymes.

The antioxidants have also been found to play a protective role against heart disease. Both vitamins C and E inhibit LDL oxidation and reduce platelet adhesion. Reduced angina and myocardial infarction have been noted with increased beta-carotene intake.

FIGURE 15-1
Antioxidant and Immune Enhancing Foods

Vitamin A

Fish-liver oil, meats, and animal products

Beta-Carotene (Vitamin A precursor)

Leafy, dark green vegetables and yellow and orange vegetables and fruits including carrots, sweet potatoes, broccoli, spinach, collard, turnip, beet, and mustard greens, kale, cantaloupe, papayas, and apricots

Vitamin C

Fruits and vegetables, especially citrus fruits, cantaloupe, kiwi, honeydew melon, pomegranate, persimmon, broccoli, greens, tomatoes, and green peppers

Vitamin E

Whole grains, vegetable oils, leafy dark greens, sweet potatoes, and organ meats

Vitamin B-6

Whole grains, leafy dark greens, potatoes, and nuts

Vitamin B-12

Fish, dairy products, organ meats, eggs, beef, and pork

Folic Acid

Leafy dark greens, legumes, and salmon

Calcium

Dairy products, leafy dark greens, salmon, tofu, and fortified soy milk

Copper

Organ meats, seafood, nuts, legumes, and fruits

Iron

Meat, poultry, fish, leafy dark greens, dried fruit, and blackstrap molasses

Magnesium

Seafood, dark green vegetables, dairy products, and whole grains

Manganese

Whole grains, nuts, leafy dark greens, organ meats, shellfish, and milk

Selenium

Broccoli, mushrooms, cabbage, celery, cucumbers, onions, garlic, brewer's yeast, grains, fish, and organ meats

Zinc

Whole grains, brewer's yeast, wheat bran and germ, sunflower seeds, seafoods, and meat

Heart Helpers

Foods rich in antioxidants such as Vitamins C and E are also good for the prevention of heart disease. Omega-3 fatty acids, or EPAs (eicosopentaenoic acids) have also been shown to have heart health benefits such as the prevention of LDL oxidation, blood clots, coronary artery spasms, and coronary artery blockages.

EPAs are found in fish oils, soybean products such as tofu, seaweed, whole grains, and beans. Cold saltwater fish such as salmon, mackerel, and herring are particularly high in EPAs, and tuna and sardines are other good sources. Try to eat fish that is caught outside coastal waters to minimize the risk of contamination with heavy metals, pesticides, and chlorinated hydrocarbons. EPAs are also available in capsule form, although most authorities agree that consuming fish is more beneficial than consuming the supplements.

Oat bran or rolled oats, taken consistently on a daily basis, lower both total cholesterol and LDL levels. Recent studies reveal that this effect can be achieved by eating either two ounces of oat bran or three ounces of oatmeal daily. The soluble fiber beta-D glucosan in oats is the responsible factor. Other sources of soluble fiber such as beans, pectin, and psyllium also lower cholesterol.

Garlic—A Super Food

Garlic has been popular as a food, a spice, and a folk medicine for thousands of years in all parts of the world. Recent scientific interest has led to a better understanding of the diverse healing properties of the "stinking rose." The National Library of Medicine lists more than 100 papers published since 1983 on garlic.

The healing properties of garlic are quite astounding—antibiotic, immune-stimulating, hypolipidemic, antihypertensive, antitumor, antihepatotox, decongestant, antiprotozoal, and insecticidal.

Raw garlic kills bacteria and boosts immune function, while cooked garlic lowers blood cholesterol, thins the blood, and acts as a decongestant. It is generally recommended that people eat about two cloves a day, both raw and cooked.

FOODS THAT HARM

The converse of a healthy diet is one that is high in fat and protein and low in complex carbohydrates. In addition, specific foods are detrimental to the proper functioning of the body.

Sugars

Unlike complex carbohydrates, which are digested steadily and slowly, sugars are digested rapidly, creating a sudden burst of energy due to a rapid rise in blood sugar levels. However, a rapid decline soon follows the peak, often resulting in fatigue, drowsiness, or nervousness. Long term sugar consumption creates chronic stress on the pancreas and promotes tooth decay.

The body reacts the same to all sugars: white sugar, corn syrup, maple syrup, or honey. Some research indicates that fructose may be metabolized at a slower pace than the other sugars. In general, it is best to limit sugar intake and to dilute fruit juices with water to a 50% concentration.

Chemical Additives

Most factory produced foods have chemical additives of one type or another. These chemicals add to the shelf-life of foods, but they are not beneficial to the body. Some have been found to be carcinogenic in animal studies performed under the auspices of the Delaney Clause of the Food, Drug, and Cosmetic Act.

Avoid additives whenever possible. In general, stay away from any food containing artificial sweeteners, artificial coloring, flavor enhancers, or sodium nitrite or nitrate.

Caffeine

Moderate intake of coffee (five to six cups a day) has been linked to increased risk of heart disease. Some research has also shown a relationship between caffeine consumption and fibrocystic breast disease, while other studies show no such relationship. Caffeine does stimulate the sympathetic nervous system, increasing adrenalin and other stress hormones. It is also vitamin depleting and is addictive for some people.

It is best to avoid or limit your intake of caffeine beverages and foods such as coffee, nonherbal teas, colas, cocoa, and chocolate products. Herbal teas, in a wide variety of flavors, and grain beverages are good hot drink substitutes. If you are tired, rather than drink a cup of coffee, try bellows breathing or yoga — the *Shoulder Stand* or a quick round of *Sun Salutation*.

Alcohol

Consumption of alcohol depletes the body's store of B-complex vitamins and, over time, has a toxic effect on the heart and liver. Those who consume even one alcoholic beverage a day have been shown to double their risk of stroke, when compared with nondrinkers, and female moderate drinkers have been found to be substantially more at risk for breast cancer. Cirrhosis, pancreatitis, hypertension, malnutrition, cardiac arrhythmias, cardiomyopathy, and breast cancer are all linked to heavy drinking.

Recent studies have shown a positive relationship between longevity and the consumption of one or two ounces of alcohol daily. These studies, however, did not examine the issue of social support, which in itself may be responsible for or contribute to increased longevity. Participants in these studies who did not drink often chose not to drink because they were not in good health or because they were recovering alcoholics. Looking at the risks versus the potential benefits of alcohol consumption, it seems advisable to limit your intake of alcoholic beverages.

Processed Baked Goods

Processed baked goods are a common source of hidden saturated fats. Many packaged cookies and pastries contain palm, cottonseed, coconut, or partially hydrogenated oils. These products also contain sugars and refined flours.

Salt

Recent evidence shows that salt is not as important a contributing factor to elevated blood pressure as was previously believed. The majority of people who have hypertension are not sensitive to salt and are able, like those without hypertension, to excrete any excess. The addition of small amounts of salt to your food is probably harmless if you are not sensitive to salt.

FOOD ROTATION

Since no single food contains all nutrients, it is important to eat a wide variety of foods to ensure that your body is properly nourished.

There is also another important reason to vary your food intake. Each food requires a unique combination of the enzymes synthesized by the body if it is to be completely digested and eliminated. If you eat the same foods day after day, year after year, your enzyme production becomes impaired, causing allergic reactions due to malabsorption. This, in turn, leads to mutation of the white blood cells, and ultimately, immune system stress. The most common food allergies are to wheat and orange juice, two staple foods of the typical American breakfast.

It takes the body seven days to replenish its store of an enzyme. Eating a given food no more than once a week thus enhances enzyme reproduction and the maintenance of a strong immune system. The digestion of sprouted foods, which contain an abundance of enzymes, does not depend on the body's synthesis of enzymes, so such foods may be consumed on a daily basis without any adverse effect.

FOOD SUPPLEMENTS

The Recommended Daily Allowances (RDAs) are the levels of intake of essential nutrients considered by the Food and Nutrition Board of the National Academy of Sciences and the Food and Drug Administration (FDA) to be adequate to meet the nutritional needs of the average healthy person. Ideally, you should be able to obtain all the nutrients you need by eating a balanced and healthful diet.

Unfortunately, the foods we eat may not be as nourishing as they should be. Grown on depleted soil with toxic fertilizers and pest repellents, much of the food in supermarkets lacks important nutrients. Comparing the taste of a supermarket tomato to an organically grown one will give you a kinesthetic experience of this reality.

Considerable loss of nutrients also takes place during the processing and preparation of foods. Lifestyle factors such as stress, pollution, strenuous exercise, pregnancy, coffee and alcohol consumption, illness, and prescription medications may all increase an individual's nutritional requirements.

Daily Supplementation

Based on the factors just described, it is advisable to support your daily diet with a nutritional supplement containing ample proportions of the antioxidants, vitamins A, C, and E, the B-complex vitamins, beta-carotene, and minerals. To maximize utilization, select supplements free from common allergens such as wheat, corn, yeast, milk, egg, or soy.

Crisis Supplementation

The need for B-complex and C vitamins increases when you are under stress. Adding these supplements to your diet can be very useful. Some formulations, specifically designed for stressful times, contain both the B-complex and C in one tablet.

Several supplements are helpful in warding off colds and flus, particularly if taken at the first sign or symptom. Perhaps the best known is Vitamin C. Zinc stimulates an effective immune response against bacteria and viruses. The combination of two American herbs, *echinacea angustifolia* and goldenseal, natural antibiotics and antivirals, is particularly potent in quickly stimulating the immune system to resist infection. The Chinese herbs licorice root and astragalus are another efficacious, natural way to combat infections.

SELECTED BIBLIOGRAPHY

Carper, J. *The Food Pharmacy: Dramatic New Evidence That Food Is Your Best Medicine.* New York: Bantam Books, 1988.

Dunne, L. J. *Nutrition Almanac*, 3rd ed. New York: McGraw-Hill, 1990.

Hendler, S. S. *The Doctors' Vitamin and Mineral Encyclopedia.* New York: Simon and Schuster, 1990.

Prevention Magazine. *Prevention's Top 100 Diet and Healing Foods: What to Eat to Defeat Disease and Peel Off the Pounds.* Emmaus, PA: Rodale Press, Inc., 1991.

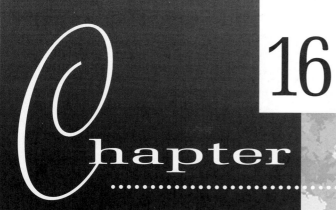

Chapter 16

Nutritional Tips and Tricks

STRESSFUL VERSUS STRESSLESS EATING

Some ways of eating are less stressful on the body than are others. Eating many different foods at one sitting is very stressful on the body, since each food requires a specific set of enzymes and each type of food requires a different pH for proper digestion. The "buffet belches" are a result of too many incomplete digestive reactions occurring at the same time. Consuming fewer foods at one time is best. If your digestion is upset or sluggish, eating only one food for the entire day can bring relief. Apples or grapes are good for this purpose, as both have a neutral pH.

COMBINING FOODS

Taking this concept one step further, certain combinations of food types have been found to be conducive to efficient digestion while others are not.

Vegetables are best combined with protein or starches; protein and starches should not be combined. A meat and potato meal or a fish and rice meal results in an acid pH for digesting the starch, which suppresses the HCl secretion necessary for digesting protein. The result is incomplete protein digestion, intestinal putrefaction, and congested lymphatics.

Fruits are best eaten uncombined with any other food. When combined with proteins or starches, their digestion is slowed, resulting in putrefaction and gas. Both citrus fruits and melons should be eaten alone, not in combination with other fruits. Citrus has an alkaline effect on the body, while melons take longer to break down and tend to create gas. Consult Figure 16-1 for a summary of foods that combine well and those that do not.

FIGURE 16-1
Food Combination Chart

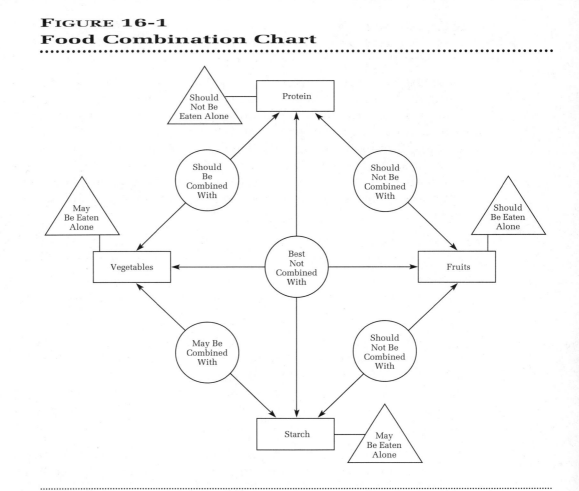

FASTING

Fasting is abstinence from solid foods or from all foods for a specified time period. There are many different types of fasts. Some permit intake of vegetable juices, others allow fruit juices, still others permit a combination of liquid ingredients, and some allow water only. A one-day fast is designed to relieve organ congestion, while more extensive fasts are geared toward deep detoxification of the body tissues.

One-Day Fasts

The secretions of the pancreas and liver are essential for the proper digestion of all foods. If these organs are weakened by congestion, they do not function efficiently. Many nutritional experts recommend that you routinely fast one day a week on apple juice, diluted by 50% with water. This strategy allows you to maintain an adequate blood sugar level while giving your organs a rest and is a particularly useful type of fast if you have overeaten or eaten fatty foods.

If fasting for a day is not convenient or has no appeal for you, there are a couple of alternatives for maintaining healthy liver function. Drinking a glass of water daily with the juice of one lemon or with a tablespoon of black cherry concentrate and an ounce of chlorophyll will enhance liver efficiency.

Extended Fasts

An extended fast—one of more than three days—results in *autolysis*, the body's digestion of its own toxins. The substances decomposed in this way are diseased, damaged, or dead cells and tissues, and fat deposits. The brain, nervous system, glands, vital organs, and essential tissues are not digested during a fast.

Extended fasts have been found useful in helping a variety of conditions including intestinal disorders, skin problems, arthritis, and cancer. Some people routinely fast with the changing of the season simply to cleanse and rejuvenate the body.

Regardless of whether you choose a water or juice fast, three things are necessary for a successful experience. First, the body must be prepared by eating very lightly, usually just vegetables, for a few days prior to the initiation of the fast. Second, you need to provide some assistance to the bowels during the fast, in the form of herbal laxatives or enemas, to release the toxins that are being broken down within the body. Third, the fast must be broken as carefully as it is initiated, usually by limiting the diet to steamed vegetables only for three days.

It is not unusual to feel tired, cold, or toxic during the first few days. These feelings usually give way to abundant energy and clarity of thought as the fast proceeds. If you are undertaking an extended fast for the first time, it is advisable to do so under the guidance of a holistic practitioner experienced with the process.

KNOWING WHAT YOU ARE EATING

Your goals for healthy eating are to avoid sugar, artificial additives, and chemicals, and to limit fat and protein. Become a careful label reader. Both promotional packaging and labels can be deceiving.

For example, many product claims are made about "no cholesterol." However, when you read the label, you will find that the product is high in saturated fat, which gets converted by your body into cholesterol. Many processed baked goods such as crackers, cookies, and so forth, often with "no cholesterol" package labels, contain saturated or hydrogenated oils.

Low-fat milk, which claims to be 2% fat, is another example of misleading packaging. The 2% actually refers to the weight of the fat content, which in actuality accounts for 32% of the product's calories. For helpful insight into how to calculate a given food's fat content, refer to Figure 16-2.

FIGURE 16-2
Calculating Food Fat Content

$$\frac{\text{Grams of fat} \times 9 \text{ calories/gram} \times 100}{\text{Total calories in food}} = \frac{\text{Percentage of calories}}{\text{from fat in food}}$$

Example: Low-fat (2%) Milk

$$\frac{5 \text{ grams of fat} \times 9 \text{ calories/gram} \times 100}{140 \text{ calories}} = 32\% \text{ fat}$$

Calories/gram: fat = 9, carbohydrates = 4, protein = 4

FDA Food Labeling Requirements

To address the issue of misleading food labels, the FDA has recently released food labeling rules and regulations to comply with the mandate of the Nutrition Labeling and Education Act of 1990.

For the first time, food producers are required to present uniform information about serving sizes and nutrients. The package information must also specify what percentage of the recommended FDA Daily Values are contained in the food. The FDA Daily Values are based on a 2,000 calorie intake comprised of 60% carbohydrates, 10% protein, 30% or less from fat, and no more than 10% from saturated fat. Daily Values are also established for cholesterol, sodium, and dietary fiber. These values are summarized in Figure 16-3.

FIGURE 16-3
FDA Daily Values

Total Fat	Less than 65 gm
Saturated Fat	Less than 20 gm
Cholesterol	Less than 300 mg
Sodium	Less than 2,400 mg
Total Carbohydrates	300 gm
Total Protein	50 gm

Although the FDA Daily Values are a step in the right direction, they are still based on a maximum of 30% fat, whereas current recommendations for prevention and reversal of degenerative disease indicate that only 10% to 15% of daily calorie intake should be from fat.

Also, it is important to be aware that the FDA regulations are not applicable to restaurant menus nor to the advertising of food products.

REACHING AND MAINTAINING YOUR IDEAL WEIGHT

More than 30 million adult Americans are overweight, and many turn to nationally advertised weight loss programs for assistance. Although some people have results in the short run, after five years more than 90% of the participants in these restricted intake programs have gained back the weight they initially lost.

Why Dieting Can Make You Fat

Dieting can actually make you gain weight. On a restricted diet, your metabolic rate goes down. The body burns calories at a slower rate because it is protecting itself from starvation. Thus when you return to your previous eating pattern after a diet, your body's slower rate of metabolism will make you tend to gain weight.

The first weight lost when dieting is from water and glycogen depletion. The body will then shed both fat and muscle, with a sedentary person losing more muscle than an active person. When you gain the weight back, water and glycogen are replaced first. If you are sedentary, you will next gain back the fat without rebuilding the lost muscle tissue. The result is an increase in the proportion of fat in your body, and a body with a higher proportion of fat burns calories less efficiently than one with a more muscular composition.

An Alternative to Dieting

The best way to reach and maintain your ideal weight is by eating a diet high in complex carbohydrates and low in fat and protein, exercising, and drinking an adequate supply of water.

Complex Carbohydrates as Your Mainstay

Complex carbohydrates have less than half the calories of fat, are digested steadily, and supply sufficient fiber for regular elimination.

Dietary fat is readily stored in the body as fat, whereas turning carbohydrates into fat requires a number of chemical reactions and the expenditure of a large amount of energy to complete them. Also, eating complex carbohydrates stimulates the sympathetic nervous system and the thyroid, resulting in more efficient metabolism.

Exercise

Regular aerobic exercise increases the body's metabolic rate and the burning of calories. Exercise also builds muscle, and a more muscular body is a more efficient metaboliser than is a less muscular one.

Water

As discussed in Chapter 14, drinking eight glasses of water a day assists in weight loss by promoting excretion of excess sodium and retained water and facilitating efficient functioning of the kidneys and liver. Drinking a couple of glasses of water an hour before each meal is a good weight loss strategy, as doing so will cause a feeling of fullness.

Be Proactive When You Eat

Be proactive rather than reactive when you eat. You can make an active choice about how you respond to food, just as you do with every other stimulus in your life. Make choices about food and eating based on values rather than on conditioned reactions or impulses. If you pause and consider the values of health, well-being, and feeling good about your appearance, these factors may help you to make eating choices that are appropriate for your values.

Envision Yourself Thin

See yourself the size you want to be. Use visualizations and affirmations to reinforce this image. Bring yourself at your ideal weight into the present with your mind.

NEW ADDITIONS TO YOUR PANTRY

Learning and incorporating new ways may take a little doing. Here are some ideas to assist you in the move toward a high complex carbohydrate and low fat and protein eating style.

Seaweed for Beans

Many people have trouble with flatulence after eating beans. By cooking beans with seaweed (a 6" strip of *kombu*), the structure of the bean is altered in such a way that it does not create gas. Just discard the seaweed after the beans are cooked.

Dairy Substitutes

If you decide to cut dairy products out of your diet, there are soy cheeses available that melt like dairy cheeses. Dairy-like beverages and ice cream-like frozen desserts made from either soy or rice, along with soy cheeses, are usually stocked in health food stores.

An easy, tasteful, and healthy substitute for cream-based soups is the use of white potatoes as a base. Simply cook the potatoes with another vegetable such as broccoli or spinach and put them in a blender or food processor until they reach a creamy consistency. The result is a nondairy cream of broccoli or cream of spinach soup. Incidentally, cooked yams or sweet potatoes seasoned with curry make another tasteful, creamy soup.

Sprouts and Sprouted Breads

Seeds are the source of all protein, fat, carbohydrates, vitamins, and minerals for the plant-to-be. Enzymes released in the sprouting process convert the protein into amino acids, the carbohydrates into simple sugars, and the fats into fatty acids. Sprouts are an easily digestible food source richer in vitamins and minerals than the plant they might have become.

Just about any seed can be sprouted. It is an easy and inexpensive process to do yourself. Otherwise, you can usually find alfalfa sprouts in the supermarket and a wider variety of sprouts in health food stores.

Highly nutritious breads made completely of sprouts, with no flour, are also available. These sprouted, unleavened breads, most commonly found in health food stores, are made of fermented grain sprouts and baked slowly at a low temperature. They are naturally sweet due to the maltose released during the fermentation process and come in a variety of flavors. Leavened sprouted breads, which look like standard sandwich breads, are another alternative that can sometimes be found in supermarkets. Look for the words "flourless" or "no flour" on the labels of both types of sprouted breads.

Dressings, Seasonings, and Sweeteners

There are a number of no-fat salad dressings on the market, some better tasting than others. Rice, balsamic, and other vinegars along with lemons and limes make a refreshing light dressing.

A variety of herbal seasonings, some with salt and some without, are available. You may also want to make your own blends.

If your "sweet tooth" just will not go away, the least harmful sweeteners are those made from natural rice or barley malt. Eating no-fat cookies and pastries sweetened with fruit juice is better than munching on the standard packaged varieties.

EATING OUT

You can adapt your new eating style to restaurant meals as well as to those served at home.

Items Available at Most Restaurants

Most restaurants will prepare a vegetable plate for you upon request. Be sure to ask that the vegetables be steamed, baked, or grilled, and prepared without oil or butter. The same instructions should be specified for fish or white meat poultry. If ordering a salad, ask that it not be dressed and request vinegar or lemon on the side. Vegetable soups are ideal as long as they are not cream-based, and baked potatoes without condiments are usually always available. Oatmeal, fresh fruits, or egg white omelets, cooked in a nonstick pan, are good breakfast choices.

Chinese Restaurants

Order steamed white rice (some restaurants now even serve brown rice) and stir-fried vegetables, with or without chicken. Request that the stir-fry be done without oil—either in water or by the "dry-wok" method. Make sure the restaurant does not add monosodium gluta-mate (MSG) to its foods, and go easy on salty soy sauce.

Italian Restaurants

Pasta with marinara or vegetable sauces and without cream, butter, or oil is a good choice. Pizza can often be ordered without cheese, topped with tomato sauce and vegetables. The minestrone or vegetable soups may be acceptable if they are not made with oil, cream, or butter. Vegetable salads, undressed and meatless, are usually available. Season with lemon or vinegar.

Mexican Restaurants

Lard is a favored ingredient in most Mexican cooking. Some restaurants are not refrying their beans, and you may be able to obtain pinto or black beans that have been cooked only in water. If this be your good fortune, a bean and rice burrito without cheese in a corn tortilla is a good choice. A dab of guacamole is acceptable, but limit the amount, as avocado is very high in fat. Ceviche, or marinated fish, often served as an appetizer in Mexican restaurants, is a good low-fat choice.

Fast Food Restaurants

If this is the only food available to you, you have to do the best you can. Try to avoid fried foods, cheeses, and sauces. Many fast food restaurants now serve baked potatoes and have salad bars with oil-free dressings or vinegar. Some of the fast food chains provide information on the nutritive content of their foods to assist you in your choices.

YOUR NUTRITIONAL PLAN

A plan is helpful when initiating any new activity. Make copies of Figure 16-4 to chart four weeks of menu planning. If you are starting from a meat-based diet, you may want to begin by including one or two vegetarian days the first week, and then adding an additional day each week for the following three weeks.

As you change your eating patterns, you may experience bloating, gas, mucus, headaches, or skin eruptions. These symptoms are quite common and are no cause for alarm. Your body is simply detoxifying and adjusting. Make sure you drink plenty of water during this time. In a week or two, you will be delighted with how much lighter and more energetic you are feeling.

FIGURE 16-4
NUTRITIONAL PLAN

	MON.	TUES.	WED.
Breakfast			
After Breakfast			
Lunch			
After Lunch			
Dinner			

THURS.	FRI.	SAT.	SUN.

SELECTED BIBLIOGRAPHY

Blauer, S. *The Juicing Book.* Garden City Park, NJ: Avery Publishing Group, 1989.

Calbon, C., and Keane, M. *Juicing For Life.* Garden City Park, NJ: Avery Publishing Group, 1992.

Cannon, G., and Einzig, H. *Dieting Makes You Fat.* New York: Simon and Schuster, 1985.

Colimore, B., and Colimore, S. S. *Nutrition & Your Body.* Los Angeles: Light Wave Press, 1978.

Johnson, J. *Road to Recovery.* Orange, CA: Joyce Johnson Wellness Center, 1990.

Mandatory Nutritional Labeling Final Rule. *Federal Register.* January 6, 1993, Vol. 58, No. 3.

Wigmore, A. *The Sprouting Book.* Wayne, IN: Avery Publishing Group, 1986.

Chapter 17

The Power
of the
Positive

CIRCUMSTANTIAL INFLUENCES

As a nurse you come in contact with many negative reactions during your typical workday. You are surrounded by patients in varying degrees of discomfort and pain. Your patients, their families, and their friends may be experiencing a wide range of negative emotions such as anger, frustration, grief, panic, fear, and hopelessness. You may also have colleagues and administrators who create less than a pleasant atmosphere around you.

CREATING A POSITIVE INTERNAL ENVIRONMENT

Your reality may be that negativity surrounds you in your daily work life and possibly in your personal life, as well. Certainly it is a good idea to change anything you can, but you may not be able to adjust all external circumstances to your liking. However, there is an important change you can make. You can create a positive and uplifting internal environment for yourself.

Creating a strong internal environment allows you to move through external negative circumstances without being brought down by them. You understand that the things happening around you are merely experiences, and that you have a choice about how you relate to those experiences.

You can choose to carry this positive environment with you at all times, everywhere you go, and into everything you do. As your internal environment becomes anchored in positivity, not only do you neutralize the negativity around you, but your presence uplifts others.

Some ways of creating this positive internal environment were addressed in Chapters 6 and 7. Here are some additional ways.

THE LAUGHTER CONNECTION

Norman Cousins, with his description of how he healed himself of an apparently "incurable" disease in *Anatomy of an Illness*, brought public attention to the power of humor and laughter as healing tools. Since then, psychoneuroimmunology researchers have documented the positive effects of laughter on the body, including increases in the number of immune cells and enhanced respiration. Laughter physically massages the internal organs, stimulates endorphin release, and increases circulation and resistive vitality against disease.

Today, many hospitals have subscribed to a service called Humor/x, a mobile cart full of humorous materials that can be wheeled into patients' rooms. Other hospitals have a special television channel that allows patients to watch comedy films at any hour. Still others have established "living room" areas, where patients can engage in a variety of cultural and artistic activities, including watching and listening to humorous material.

Humor and Stress

Canadian researchers Dr. Rod A. Martin and Dr. Herbert M. Lefcourt found that those individuals who value humor the most are most capable of coping with severe personal problems and tension (Martin & Lefcourt, Note 1). They also noted that people with the greatest ability to improvise humorous routines spontaneously were also best able to counteract stress. Other studies by psychologists Dr. Annette Goodheart and Dr. Alice M. Isen have shown the link between humor and creative problem solving ability (Leighty, Note 2 and Isen et al, Note 3).

Humor Prescription

The word humor comes from the Latin word *umere*, which means to be fluid, to flow like water. Making light of a situation or experience changes things by moving your perspective from one place to another.

Make humor and laughter a part of your life. Weave it into the tapestry of everything you do. Humor is more about a worldview or perspective than it is about any specific joke, film, or comedy routine. Taste in humor is personal; humor, itself, is universal.

EVERYONE'S A TEACHER

You have an extensive group of people in your personal orbit. Some are supportive friends. Others—patients, coworkers, supervisors, relatives—may not react or respond to you in a positive way.

Rather than allowing those who are acting in a negative way to upset or aggravate you, you can reframe how you look at them. Let yourself know that everyone is doing exactly what they personally need to be doing to learn exactly what it is they need to learn.

Instead of reacting, ask yourself, "What is this person teaching me?" or "How can I become better as a result of this experience?" For example, if a coworker is continuously making snide comments about your appearance, rather than responding with a similar nasty remark, ignore it and instead look inside.

First, look back at your recent interactions with this person and see if there is anything you might have said or done, intentionally or unintentionally, that may have generated her reaction to you. If you can identify a less than desirable behavior on your part, then perhaps a "heart-to-heart" or an apology is in order.

If not, look a little deeper. Look at the nature of her character and her interactions with others. Is she a competitive person? Is she jealous? Does she always need to be right? This analysis does take some work, but the effort will lead you to the source of the problem and the lesson in it for you.

Everyone, every interaction, and every experience is a teacher for you. Once you understand the lesson, you do not need to repeat it. Until you understand, the faces and places will change, but the lesson will remain the same. Engaging in this process assists you in building a strong internal environment.

MEDIA MASSAGE

We live in an age in which we are constantly massaged by the media—print, television, radio, movies, and so on. Much of the message of the mass culture is negative, and you are influenced by it consciously and subconsciously. But you can carefully select your channels and tune yourself in to positive media. This is yet another way for you to build a strong internal environment.

Watching the 11:00 P.M. news before you go to bed is not a good way to maintain a positive internal environment. Similarly, viewing violent movies and television programs does little for your sense of internal peace and harmony. Just as you choose positive, supportive people to be your friends, select movies, books, and magazines that uplift you.

Music is powerful. Studies performed on plants show that they flourish with classical music and wither with rock music. Similarly, you can use music to nourish yourself and strengthen your internal environment. Music therapy research reveals that soothing, relaxing music creates positive emotional neural messages, resulting in favorable modulation of the endocrine, immune, and autonomic nervous systems. Listening to such music shifts you into the right brain—that space of intuition and deep healing.

RECHARGING YOURSELF

As a nurse you are constantly in the position of giving. To continue in that mode day in and day out, you need to engage in activities that recharge you with vitality and optimism.

Some activities which can recharge you have been described in earlier chapters of this book—meditation in Chapter 7, breathing in Chapter 8, aerobic exercise in Chapter 9, and yoga in Chapter 10. Nature is a wonderful healer, and so is the circus. Make time for fun in your life. Any activity, person, or thing that brings you joy and happiness is beneficial.

Create a "good time" schedule for yourself using the chart in Figure 17-1. If you tend to put off your own enjoyment, it is particularly important that you engage in this exercise. Do at least one fun or restorative thing each day. It can be as simple as taking time to smell the flowers in the garden you pass on your way to work, taking a bubble bath, playing your favorite relaxing music, or spending time with a close friend. Plan more extended activities such as horseback riding, skating, going to the theater, or visiting an amusement park as frequently as time and resources permit.

FIGURE 17-1
Good Time Schedule

	ACTIVITY #1	ACTIVITY #2	ACTIVITY #3
Mon.			
Tues.			
Wed.			
Thurs.			
Fri.			
Sat.			
Sun.			

NOTES

1. Martin, R. A., and Lefcourt, H. M. "Sense of humor as a moderator of the relation between stressors and moods." *Journal of Personality and Social Psychology, 45* (1983):1313–1324.

2. Leighty, M. "Laughter helps the heart and soul." *The Houston Chronicle.* (June 9, 1987.)

3. Isen, A. M., Johnson, M. M. S., Mertz, E., and Robinson, G. F. "The influence of positive affect on the usualness of word associations." *Journal of Personality and Social Psychology, 48* (1985):1413–1426

SELECTED BIBLIOGRAPHY

Borysenko, J. *Fire in the Soul: A New Psychology of Spiritual Optimism.* New York: Warner Books, 1993.

Cousins, N. *Anatomy of an Illness.* New York: W.W. Norton & Co., 1979.

Cousins, N. *Head First: The Biology of Hope and the Healing Power of the Human Spirit.* New York: Penguin Books, 1989.

Dossey, B. M., and Guzzetta, C. E. "Biobehavioral interventions." In *Cardiovascular Nursing: Holistic Practice.* St. Louis: Mosby-Year Book, 1992: 100–122.

Guzzetta, C. E. "Music therapy: Nursing the music of the soul." In *Music: Physician for Times to Come.* Wheaton, IL: The Theosophical Publishing House, 1991: 146–166.

Klein, A. *The Healing Power of Humor.* Los Angeles: Jeremy P. Tarcher, 1989.

Robinson, V. *Humor and the Health Professions*, 2nd ed. Thorofare, NJ: Slack, 1991.

Chapter 18

The Changing You

Life is in a constant state of flux. Nothing remains the same. Change happens whether or not you want it to happen. But when you decide to mobilize yourself for personal change in a positive direction, you are calling upon yourself to be more. By deciding to adopt any of the new ideas or behaviors presented in the previous chapters, you have accepted the challenge to become more whole in body, mind, and/or spirit. Congratulations for your willingness and your courage.

STEP-BY-STEP

It is important to take things one step at a time and at a pace that is comfortable for you. For example, you may be comfortable making changes in your eating and exercise habits at the same time. Someone else may be overwhelmed by attempting to do both at once, whereas another person may be perfectly able to implement change in three or four areas of her life.

It is essential to know your own limits and not compare yourself with anyone else. Establish your personal goals and move toward them. Beware of taking on too much too fast. The danger in overloading is that you might decide to abandon all activities with the same rapidity and intensity with which you embraced them.

BE GENTLE WITH YOURSELF AS YOU CHANGE

Getting in Gear

If you have trouble motivating yourself to begin adopting a new habit or behavior, you may want to look at your resistance. Usually what you resist the most is what needs to be changed the most.

What is behind resistance is fear. Change can be frightening. You are looking at becoming different, at shifting from something you know to something unknown. Even though the shoes you are walking in are worn out and do not fit you any more, they have been with you for quite a while and you know them.

Do not try to force yourself to change. Just accept that your fears are surfacing and that this is where you are right now. You need to move your focus from whatever activity you are resisting—new eating patterns, meditation, and so on—to imaging the new you that would result from the activity you are resisting.

Your tools for doing this are affirmations and visualizations, bringing the new transformed you into the present (see Chapter 6). Also, doing the "Jumping Backwards" exercise from the same chapter may be extremely useful in helping you discover hidden attitudes or beliefs that are influencing your current lack of motivation.

Stalling

A different but related obstacle may challenge you. You may find that you were very motivated, made some progress, and were happy with yourself, and then suddenly, for reasons totally unknown to you, you just stopped doing what you were doing. For example, you stopped exercising, went on an eating binge, or picked a fight with a coworker.

If you do experience this, be gentle with yourself. Many times, subconscious patterns come to the surface when you begin to change. Even though consciously you are going "full steam ahead," there may be hidden beliefs or attitudes that only become activated when you are fully engaged in transforming yourself.

Work with yourself to see if you can identify the source, using mindcise exercises (see Chapter 6). If for some reason that does not work for you, just take a break. Be patient, knowing that you will pick up where you left off when you are ready.

RELEASING THE OUTDATED

Just as you clear outdated clothes out of your closet to make room for new ones, you release outdated habits, attitudes, and beliefs to make way for better ones. Sometimes the releasing process may challenge you as you find yourself very attached to your old way of being, even though it no longer serves you well.

You may find yourself feeling depressed or anxious. This is not unusual. What you are doing is mourning the death of your old ways. It is far better to feel the feelings than to suppress them. After all, these habits and beliefs were your close friends and now they are gone. It is important to remember, however, that in releasing the lesser you are making room for the greater.

CHANGING THE INNER CHANGES THE OUTER

Keeping a personal journal is a good way to track how you change, both internally and externally. It is a supportive resource and a convenient feedback tool for charting your journey toward holism.

As you become more healthy in body, mind, and spirit, your self-concept will be different, and the way your external environment responds to you will change. You may find your friends changing, you may decide to find or be offered a new job, or you may experience yourself responding emotionally in a totally fresh manner. As your internal environment becomes more integrated and stronger, your external environment reflects a more abundant and fulfilling life experience back to you.

One experience you may have as you are becoming healthier is that people who have known you for a long while still see only the "old you" and respond to that outdated image. This is more common with regard to beliefs and attitudes than to physical changes, because physical changes are much easier to see and understand. Do not let their reactions deter you from your growth. They simply do not know the "new you," or else their own fears and insecurities may prevent them from welcoming your new way of being in the world.

CONTINUING THE JOURNEY

You have begun your journey toward embracing a balance in mind, body, and spirit. You are renewing yourself and blossoming into a fuller life experience. Continue unfolding and enjoy who you are, who you are becoming, and each step on your pathway.

SELECTED BIBLIOGRAPHY

Bridges, W. *Transitions: Making Sense of Life's Changes*. Menlo Park, CA: Addison-Wesley, 1980.

Sinnetar, M. *Elegant Choices, Healing Choices*. New York: Paulist Press, 1988.

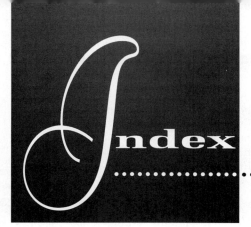

Index

RESOURCES

For information regarding in-house continuing education workshops and California mountain retreats, please contact:

Sherry Kahn, MPH
Self-Care for Caregivers
(310) 285-3245

For information regarding organizational transformation consultation, work redesign, and effective employee–employer relations, please contact:

Mileva Saulo, EdD, RN
Saulo and Associates
21116 Rose
Mission Viejo, CA 92691
(714) 830-3328